EMS 3: CAD

computer assisted despair

Semon Strobos

ISBN:1530870593
ISBN-13:9781530870592

CAD stands for computer assisted dispatch. Over the last 13 years, my job has gone from 80% patient care/20% documentation, to 20/80, reversed. Everyone in medicine complains about the same thing. Rather than write a funny book about computer frustration, I'll just use the title, and write about EMS calls.

But in passing I will mention, first, that all other equipment failures are referred to "materials management." If your cardiac monitor or your pulse oximeter don't work, you get them to deal with it. But it is your responsibility to file an ePCR (electronic patient care report, formerly "run form") on every patient by the end of shift. If the computer fails to assist you in this noble endeavor, that is your problem.

Second, I once watched an MIT computer engineer spend 20 minutes attempting to buy a tram ticket at a terminal, including using two different credit cards, while 3 trams went by. He finally took the fourth, without a ticket. After he explained his situation to the conductor, the man issued him a special card designed exactly for this, clearly common, occurrence.

Semon Strobos

Glossary

Your best bet is to use Google, or if you're in Kindle, tap the word or abbreviation you want to know more about. Wiki has good material on most of the below too.

A Fib: atrial fibrillation
AMS: altered mental status
BVM: bag valve mask or ambu-bag
Bi-pap: A C-Pap with two settings, one for exhale, one for inhale
Brady: bradycardia
Cardiovert: shock a malign rhythm to restore normal sinus rhythm
C-pap: continuous positive airway pressure delivery device.
COPD : chronic obstructive pulmonary disease
CHF: congestive heart failure
DC: discontinue, disconnect
D stick: blood sugar
ED: emergency department
EMS: emergency medical service
EMT: emergency medical technician, either Basic or Paramedic
ER: emergency room, same as ED
ET: endotracheal tube
GCS: Glasgow coma score
HTN: hypertension
ICU: intensive care unit
IV: intravenous or intravenous line
LOC: loss of consciousness
MI: myocardial infarct, heart attack
MOI: mechanism of injury
MVA: motor vehicle accident
NRB: nonrebreather mask, ambu-bag
PE: pulmonary embolism
SAT: oxygen saturation
V Fib: ventricular fibrillation
V tach: ventricular tachycardia

CONTENTS

HOW TO HURT PATIENTS

Every call is a story. They all have a beginning, a crisis or problem, development, some kind of resolution or failure to resolve, which is the same thing in a story, even if the two are profoundly different in real life, and then there's an ending. Usually you don't know how it's all going to turn out finally for the patient, but most stories don't resolve everything either.

The calls that don't work out tend to stick in my mind. There are many reasons for that besides traumatic shock. In the first place, there's never been a perfect call. There's always something you could have done better or quicker; there's always some unanticipated problem that at the very least slowed you down.

The ones that worked out more or less according to the textbook aren't very memorable, unless something dramatic happened. You don't remember brushing your teeth except for the time you poked yourself in the eye or couldn't find the toothpaste.

Also, you review stuff, and if everything went well, there's not much to review.

The interesting thing for this chapter and the next one is that if you follow the protocols, then even calls where you spin your wheels, or don't get to do what you want to do, still often work out well for the patient. That's how the protocols are designed. They are redundant, like airplane design, or the human body. If one system fails there's backup.

I like to start these books with something more dramatic so I'll start with three calls where I hurt patients, two of them deliberately.

After the accidental one, my boss said that in 18 years as a paramedic she had never hurt a patient. She's an honest person generally, but either she doesn't remember, she's not telling the truth for some instructional purpose, or she had 18 years of pussy calls.

This time we pushed the stretcher around a corner into a dialysis center and my new partner was pushing too hard. She tended to push too hard quite a bit, so my intention was to let the stretcher bang into the doorway gently to teach her to back off a bit. I hadn't calculated on how tall this patient was, though, and it happened his foot was sticking out just at the point of impact.

The weight of stretcher and patient is substantial. You have to watch elbows particularly. You can get impressive impact on very frail body parts.

This time the impact was very light. I was intending there to be just a tiny collision, enough to get her attention, rather than a big bang. Still, given how frail this paralyzed and kidney-less patient was, he bruised his big toe slightly. By the time we took off his sock and looked, there was no bleeding, but there was a small wound right under the toe nail.

And of course the main problem here is that a bedbound diabetic patient can't heal well. The other problem was that his wife was a harridan. Even when his transport went perfectly, she was never satisfied.

I asked her to help with his feet once, just to guide them gently so there would be less twisting on his legs, and she told me that she didn't do that, the nurse did.

"Yes, ma'am," I said, and got the nurse.

I asked her to sign for him, as he was blind, and she said the same thing.

"Yes, ma'am."

So my boss had a problem I wish I had not handed her.

Things happen. In 11 years of moving patients who are heavy and awkward into and around places not designed for moving patients, on rare occasions things will not go gracefully even if you are conscientious and patient. People who are injured, sick, or obese do not merely suffer from those conditions. They suffer from our efforts to help them, which do not work as well as they do with people in better shape and more normal circumstances.

We were assigned to transport that same patient on his next dialysis, Wednesday following.

I called the dispatcher. "Is that wise?" I said. "I mean, have you seen *The Lost World* or *Jurassic Park*? Remember when the hero, whatsisname, asks the paleontologist if the T Rex is going to remember him from the time he messed with her baby? I mean, am I going to get the same reaction? Is the T Rex going to say, "YOU!"

We transported without incident. T Rex was off in the primeval forest somewhere bellowing at someone else.

But there were two other, much more dramatic calls where I deliberately hurt patients. You had to be there. And you will be, just listen.

We rolled up to a rollover on I 35. It was a funky old truck with no roof. Or actually the roof had been sheared off. The truck was lying on its driver's side. In the driver's seat was the driver, a young guy, maybe 18. He was just sitting there, kind of on his left side. If you took a picture and held it the right way it would look like he was just calmly sitting in the normal driver's position.

I got the second, Basic, crew and the firemen first responders to continue extricating him onto a back board, with my c-collar already in place. I learned later that they just asked him to crawl out and lie on the board, which was absolutely not the way they were supposed to do it. It would have been hard, moving him out onto a back board, but there were four of them and it was their job. And one they were trained to do.

Still, he came out fine and the reason I was not there to supervise the extrication was that Cliff and I were busy with our second patient.

She was the driver's Mom. They had been driving back from a party, both drunk. I seem to remember it was Christmas. New Year's Eve? We found her on the other side of the truck, by the upended wheels. At first we thought she was dead. The truck had rolled over her and crushed her into the ground.

Then we saw her breathing.

Our first problem was making sure the truck didn't right itself and fall back down onto us and the patient while we were working her. We got firemen to start on stabilizing the truck and told them to warn us if anything moved so we could get out of the way.

We didn't feel we had time to wait until they were done before getting to work, even though you are supposed to wait until a scene is safe. This rule is because getting injured yourself doesn't help at all. More patients, fewer medics, But "the platinum ten minutes" means you should try to get a severely injured patient in route within ten minutes, so they can arrive at definitive care well within "the golden hour" people tend to have, after severe trauma, before organ systems crash.

Cliff was telling me even before he took vitals that we couldn't get her out of the ground without hurting her further.

"So what do we do?" I said. "Leave her here? Wait till a trauma surgeon and a paleontologist arrive to dig her out? We gotta move her."

All the correct protocols about log rolling her onto a backboard, not manipulating her neck at all when putting on her cervical collar, could not be followed as closely as we would have liked, because she was buried like a dinosaur fossil. If we had had several weeks instead of ten minutes, and paleontological instead of EMT training, we could have gotten her out totally unhurt and intact, using those little brushes and dental tools paleontologists use.

We did the best we could. It wasn't too bad either. She came out considerably easier than a fossil. And we did get her to Wilford Hall trauma center alive and still breathing, with decent vitals, IV en route, according to Hoyle. She was partially conscious, moaning sometimes, and with some reflexes. But we definitely did hurt her getting her out of the dirt, and we may have aggravated some of the fractures she undoubtedly had.

I talked to the son driver before I left the ER. He asked about his Mom, which was his chief concern. He was still in decent shape. Medically. The best I could tell him was that she was still breathing. He started crying. I kind of hope they didn't charge him for vehicular homicide. DUI.

The third and last in this series is one of the more chaotic calls I had. Though so many of them are controlled chaos of one kind or another. This was another rollover, again with an ejection. It's funny how in the 50's people used to say,

"Fortunately, he was thrown clear of the wreck," when we now know that ejection is the worst possible MOI. Though, as badly constructed as cars were in those days, sometimes being thrown clear might have been better than being impaled on the rigid steering column, or sheered by windshield fragments, or crushed by engine components breaching the cabin.

I was with Rod instead of Cliff this time. Rod was ex Special Forces and had weathered his deployments pretty well for the most part. He had an impressive presence, real gravitas, and was well spoken enough so that his previous job had been as a radio announcer. He was close to 50 but had recently married a 20 something, which impressed everyone, until he found her with another guy, and packed up and left for another state, where he went back to radio. He wasn't my partner very long because I did not talk enough. He needed conversation and companionship when posted, which is reasonable enough. It can be a long lonely shift those days when you spend 24 hours at the station, or posted, with few or no calls.

I need reading matter, myself. Some peace and quiet at least some of the time. I've always been much addicted to my own company.

The other problem which came up during our tenure together was after a call for a Spanish-only tree surgeon who fell out of a tree. I cut all his clothes off him to look for injuries, which the firemen first responders didn't like, but that is what you do. They knew better than to say anything on scene.

We were ready to roll out and one of the women fire crew was refusing to hand over his documents. "Just a minute, I'm almost done," she said.

Some volunteers get assigned to documentation, so the fire department gets paid. Sometimes they volunteer for that chore because they don't feel comfortable with patient contact or fire suppression. Maybe they have a boyfriend among the crew and want to be part of the enterprise without getting bloody or burned. Well, more power to them. Paperwork is godly. Or at least immutable. But sometimes they may take their assignment too seriously. They get to be like the librarian who doesn't want anyone to touch the books or take them out of the library. If they miss some info they can always call our station later to get it. They should not be holding up transport.

Rod was livid. He considered this, not only insubordination, but in effect refusing a direct order under fire. So when the fire chief called us later about something else, he was kind of expecting a friendly apology of sorts from me. Rod had snatched the papers and shoved her out of the way.

"I know people get a little wound up on scene sometimes," the chief said. "No hard feelings. Rod's a good guy."

"No," I said. "You don't really get it. Tell your crew never to hold up transport for any reason, much less paperwork. You have to understand, Rod is Special Forces. He saw it as refusing a direct order during combat. You have to understand, Andy, in Iraq, in that situation, he would've just pulled out his service revolver and put a round in Becky's head."

Andy didn't say anything.

But at this later call, what Rod and I found on this accident scene was a 21 year old male in a wrecked and overturned pickup, and a 34 year old female about ten feet from it.

8

The male was in pretty good shape, as someone will be who has been in an MVA with his seatbelt on. Rod and I left him to the Basic truck.

The female, not so good. She was alert and oriented, stable vitals, good color, but she also had multiple displaced fractures in her lower body. We suspected fx pelvis, hips, tib/fib and even femurs.

She was dressed in a little black dress, half torn off her, and black lace underwear, ditto. We learned later from the Basics who had talked to the driver that he had been leaving a bar when she drove up, and she ended up in his truck with him. The wreck had been caused by her pulling his dick out of his pants in route, and that was why she wasn't in a seat belt.

So here we have this hot number, half naked, the clothes half torn off her, beautiful café au lait skin, and a lot of it, and a gang of men around her with their hands on her. Furthermore, she is pleading "Don't touch me, no, don't move me, wait, just wait a minute" because of the pain we were causing her by attempting to log roll her onto backboard without causing further injury. She is saying no, but we are not obeying.

In theory, because she was alert and oriented, she could decline care altogether and stay there lying in the field until she bled to death from internal injuries. But she was clearly hysterical and she was not declining care. She was just asking us to wait.

Again, we will pause if we have to move an injured person, give them a moment to compose themselves, take a deep breath or whatever, but that's in a case where waiting isn't putting her very life at risk. What we were determined and intent on, despite anything she said, was getting her safely packaged and in route to a level one trauma center in as close to the platinum ten minutes as we could manage.

But it still would have looked like some kind of theatrical rape scene to a camera. Half naked, sexily clad woman whimpering no, men palpating her, doing a rapid trauma exam to locate injuries, holding her down, tying her down, in effect, as we duct taped her to the backboard, and all this despite her expressed wishes. Taking no not to mean no.

There's no doubt that we hurt her doing this, and also no doubt in my mind that we saved her life.

There was this momentary erotic thrill like a passing cloud. It was not a sexual thing, exactly. I have to get some help here from William Carlos Williams and Freud to explain it better. Freud said that the erotic drive is much larger than just a sexual drive. It encompasses pretty much every forward impulsive physical feeling a person has for another person. This woman was kind of out of shape and had a bit of a belly on her, so while I wouldn't say she was unattractive, she wasn't some kind of knockout I would be bowled over by under more normal circumstances. And these were not normal circumstances. We were streaming adrenaline, not testosterone, in a driven rush to follow our training and rescue her. Adrenaline is fight or flight, not testosterone, which is feed or breed. Opposite parasympathetic hormones.

Adrenaline makes your hands shake. I always had to disguise my trembling hands from patients or family or crew members as I was starting an IV in an emergency. Somehow the shaking does not impair your coordination. It doesn't seem to impede your focus or decision making, nor make you forget your training.

Although it can. People can panic or get tunnel vision. Mostly newbies, but Homer says even the greatest heroes are subject to Panic Fear at times. No man is more powerful than the god. Pan. Though Homer records no worse than caution for Achilles, the greatest of heroes. Homer felt people don't really have immortal souls or immutable characters, just tendencies, which circumstances and social settings can over-rule.

But more usually "fear of death just wonderfully focusses the mind." Like Napoleon, you shoot one admiral "pour encourager les autres." Still, you don't like to let people around you see that the medic in charge has uncontrollably shaking hands.

William Carlos Williams, the New Jersey Poet and Doctor, wrote a short story about a young girl he had to examine for diphtheria. She was wild, out of control, gorgeous, untamable, behaving like some beautiful wild animal. She was determined not to let him see her throat. Williams describes a titanic struggle in which, in a kind of holy rage, he attacked the little girl, determined to subdue and defeat her at any cost. He had to see her throat. If her airway was swelling closed, she would die without interventions. He succeeded. He was honest and perceptive enough to describe the exam as an erotic assault, in the Freudian sense, with the doctor almost as out of control as his feral patient.

This was something like that. We were determined to dominate this woman, bend her to our will, despite what she was saying. We felt no more than pity for her pleas. We were absolutely convinced, not only that this was the right thing to do, without any shadow of doubt, but that it was what she really wanted us to do, despite what she was saying, and that she would look back on this, if she remembered it at all, with gratitude. But it still felt and looked kind of like a rape scene in a blue movie. Nobody said anything or did anything or touched her anywhere except for what was purely professional and necessary, but I suspect I was not the only one who was having this weird echo.

URBAN MYTHS

There are two EMS stories that every medic hears, which I actually have come to believe are myths passed down the generations. They always occurred to some other medic in some other district, or someone heard about them from someone else. They never happened to the medic telling the story, nor was he an actual witness.

The first is that a medic gets fired for bringing in a trauma patient to a level one trauma center with an impaled object he has failed to find and report.

The impaled object is a vibrator and it is "impaled" exactly where you would expect it to be impaled.

Now, technically, that might qualify as impaled, but that is not what we mean by impaled, is it? An impaled object, by the way, has to be carefully stabilized in place, and the patient transported without removing it. This is because it may be tamponading a blood vessel, or otherwise more dangerous to remove than to leave alone. The exceptions are when the impaled object impinges on the airway or impedes CPR. There are true stories of patients being impaled on fence palliers or finials and construction people with plasma cutters having to remove a section of the fence rather than a crew removing the patient from it.

The second tall tale concerns a motor vehicle accident in which a male patient has lost a goodly chunk of his penis, which is then found severed in a woman patient's mouth, owing to her having been in the process of performing oral sex at the time the accident occurred.

I guess this is possible and could have happened somewhere some time but it's been passed down so far and so long that its origins may be in a Roman chariot race.

VAL

Val Criado is a fit, elegant 50ish Hispanic male whom it was my honor and pleasure to work with as a partner. I say elegant because in the traditions of his macho culture it is possible to be very masculine and at the same time concerned with your appearance and that of everyone around you. He wore several silver Navaho style rings, a nice haircut, and carried skin moisturizer around with him, which he would hand to me when he felt my skin looked too dry, along with advising me when I needed a haircut or a nose hair trim. He was in the habit of getting up every morning at 6, spending an hour or more in the gym before his 9 o clock, 12 hour shift. The warm up alone of his weight training routine was more intense that anything I had done in a weight room since I was in my 20's. Then he would soak in the jacuzzi for a while. One days he felt his body needed some rest he would only do the jacuzzi.

He was completely bilingual but more comfortable in Spanish, in which he was pithy, articulate, slangy and really funny. He in fact did not entirely trust Anglos. He made an exception for me partly because I like tripas but mostly because he said I did not strike him as Anglo. Well, I'm Dutch. I'm honored to be an honorary Latino.

I've hardly ever met anyone with as much natural unfeigned compassion as Val. He treated his patients like family. He knew all their names, and those of everyone else in San Antonio, seemingly, including anyone on a hospital staff he had ever met.

The sole support of his family, he lived on a piece of land inherited from his family, who have been living in San Antonio from time immemorial. It's a Spanish city. Not called Saint Anthony. So, with the help of family members, he also did everything on his house and land, plumbing, digging septic tanks, roofing, raising donkeys, chickens, dogs, ducks and geese. He liked the eggs. Somewhere in San Antonio lived a family member or old friend who could help with anything required. Including, he once offered, handle a problem I might be having with a neighbor suspected of poisoning my dog.

He was accused once of kissing patients. Now, if you are thinking this was some kind of inappropriate sexual thing, that would be of course be a huge no no. I mean, we are supposed to wear gloves every time we even touch patients' sheets. But these were not attractive young women. They were elderly Mexican ladies, in their 80's and in poor health. It is the custom for an Hispanic male to address a woman of that age as "Mama." In fact, Mamacita. This is done fondly and affectionately with a kind of respect but not with any deference or obsequiousness.

"Mamacita," he would say, tucking them in on their way to dialysis, and not infrequently kissing them. "Where is your lunch? Where is your extra blanket? You know it gets cold at dialysis."

One of these mildly demented old ladies had 5 or 6 coarse hairs growing out of her chin. "Mamacita," Val said, "You know you can't go around looking like that." Then Val proceeded to pluck them out with his handsome fingers. She looked kind of stunned but pleased.

"Didn't it hurt?" the supervisor I was telling this story to said.

"Well, yes, of course. But she was grateful."

I was telling this to Sally, my boss, actually, because she was mad at Val for forgetting some equipment and having to go back for it. I was trying to show her what a fine medic he was, really, faults and all. He WOULD take his time. Also, though, move morbidly obese patients by himself, as a challenge. Besides strength, he had technique.

"Well, everyone should make sure their patients have blankets and lunch, like that," Sally said. "Think of how you would want your mom to be treated."

Hard to satisfy her.

"Yeah," I said, "but he doesn't just treat them well. They really are like family to him." Often literally. He seemed to know everyone in the city, certainly everyone he had ever met. Knew all the nurses' and techs' names. And stories.

We once took a guy from the ER to a psych facility for a suicide attempt, after he had been stabilized. Hector had made couple of really serious ones, having to be cut down from a hanging once.

This guy was getting along with Val like a house on fire. They spoke the same language, and I don't just mean Spanish. Val has had a kind of checkered past himself. He used to cat around a lot in his younger days, and get into fights in bars regularly enough so that at least one judge was familiar enough with him to threaten him with jail if he saw him again.

Our patient was a former kick boxer. He was kind of out of shape by this time but still pretty formidable. I was in the back with him when he demanded we stop at the ER, after we picked him up on the floor, to get his stuff which had been left in the ER.

I came back with his clothes but he said we were missing his wallet and boots. I want back in. They couldn't find them. This was kind of late in the shift so I was more bent on getting the call over with than patient extras, frankly.

He sent me back in to do better. Once inside I saw him coming in, following me. He had loosed itself from the stretcher and hopped out of the ambulance, followed by Val.

"You gotta try harder," Hector told me. "You can't just take their answer."

The story turned out to be that he didn't really care about the missing boots or even his wallet, but about the scarf wrapped in plastic that had belonged to his dead daughter, who had died at 2 years old of encephalitis. This was a major issue in his suicidal despondency.

"I know I should try to get over it," he said, "but I keep falling back."

He was talking to me in English but to Val in Spanish. His demeanor was getting pretty threatening. The ER charge nurse was taking him very seriously indeed by this time, sending staff to try harder.

Meanwhile Hector was on his cell phone with his sister. Most of this conversation was in Spanish but he deliberately switched to English to say, just loud enough to be heard, "if you don't hear from me in few minutes, I want you to get some bail money together and meet me down at the courthouse, because I'm about to go apeshit." I gathered this was not a new and unimaginable problem for the sister.

The head nurse summoned a security guard. He turned up shortly, all 5'6' of him. Hector looked at him briefly, slender but pudgy, turned away and said, "Well, that isn't going to slow me up much." A matter of fact judgment call.

A second security guard was sent for. She turned out to be an obese female, maybe 5'4". Hector acceded her a brief appraising glance and went back to business.

Fortunately the relic was found. Hector embraced Val, and condescended to do the same for me after I sincerely apologized for not taking his serious troubles more seriously. I admired him by this time. He had just perceptibly hesitated before affording this Anglo an abrazo. We transported without further incident and I had a good talk with him. He kept the scarf wrapped in plastic because it still smelled like his daughter. His life was a mess but his values were intact.

I had noticed Val standing calmly to the side during the high point of this drama in the ER, surveying the scene. Afterwards I asked him what was going through his mind.

"Well," he said, coolly. "I was going to defend myself, of course, but otherwise I was just going to enjoy the show." He was helpful and courageous by nature, but he didn't feel he had a dog in this fight.

THE DIVINE PROTOCOLS

We got a call for a "sick person," which can be anything. Maybe it means the call taker couldn't figure out what the chief complaint was or couldn't figure out how to describe it in EMT code. Of course any call can be anything. You don't know till you get there.

She was 88, a true sweet old lady, in a little yellow brick house with a dry lawn in an older, inexpensive suburb in our district, SW San Antonio. She was very apologetic about calling, because her only complaint was she had discovered some swellings on her head, and she was worried they might be metastases from her cancer. She had no other way of getting to her doctor, being old and sick.

While I was doing my exam, I asked if anything hurt, if she was feeling all right, had there been any changes. No findings. Lungs clear, belly soft, alert and oriented, warm pink and dry, vital signs stable, except a thready pulse.

She said she had been feeling weak. Well, of course, I thought, you have cancer and you're 89. Of course you feel weak. Still, she had some remote cardiac history, and we were a long way out, so I put her on the monitor.

Much to my surprise, she was running SVT. Supraventricular Tachycardia is a paroxysmal rhythm which comes on suddenly. It means the atrial pacemaker in the top of the heart is not running the show. Something else up there is, and it's causing the heart to run really fast. In fact faster than it can with a normal rhythm. It's a bit like a short circuit in an electrical device, which the heart is. This can mean that the ventricles don't have time to fill properly before squeezing, and so perfusion is compromised, causing for example mental status changes or low blood pressure.

If the patient is seriously symptomatic, you shock immediately. Otherwise you are supposed to get IV access in the left AC--the bend of the elbow—and slam adenosine with a saline flush chaser. Adenosine only lasts seconds in the body, so it has to go in fast, close to the heart and in full strength. If the first 6 mg doesn't work, you go on to 12 and then another 12.

People who get SVT have usually had it before. It's a chronic ailment, like asthma or anything else that keeps coming back. You can find it in people of any age, but it's more common in younger people. It can be set off by drinking coffee or by other stimulants.

Older people with a fast atrial rhythm are more likely to be in A Fib: atrial fibrillation, where the atria are just quivering. The "atrial kick" is just 10%, though, so the ventricles keep things going just fine, usually. Unless the heart responds to the fibrillation by running too fast: rapid ventricular response, RVR.

But young people can also run A Fib, like after too much partying, which is called holiday heart.

And older people can run SVT. Like my sweet old lady.

Yellow counterpane, yellow sweater, yellow brick house. My favorite color too. Cheerful, but not aggressive like red, or weird like orange or purple. We were going to get along famously.

Green is nice, nature's color, but too subdued. God is trying to keep us calm. But I get depressed enough already. So don't even talk to me about blue. Though I do like indigo.

It's complicated. I do like some blue things like jeans. Or periwinkles. Blood is crimson. Appropriate. Makes quite a statement. A medic has to be ambivalent about blood, though. It is our livelihood. We have to be in love with it. But mostly we're fighting it.

Men are not supposed to know colors. Adorable and teal are not in our language. I know the names of trees too. I like to know the names of things.

So, anyway, after this call and others like it, I now get the adenosine ready, get the IV access, and then monitor. Treat the patient not the monitor. Many patients tolerate these rhythms really well, so it's smarter just to take them to the ER than to try to cardiovert.

The operative MO is, it's better for a patient to crack after you get on scene than before you arrive; even better in the truck while you're rolling, and best of all in the emergency room. So get them there as quickly as possible, even if it's a medical "stay and play," and not a trauma "load and go." This was one of the few bones of contention I had with Cliff. He liked to hang out with the firemen on BS or clearly non-emergent scenes; I liked to get my on scene times looking respectable and get the patient rolling. Inevitably someone will crash. And then I have to deal with it in the back of the truck. He just has to drive.

What adenosine does is more or less the same as what shocking does. It stops the heart. This is kind of seriously alarming. You don't want it to stay stopped. But the idea is, it's the same as turning off your computer, then turning it back on to reboot. The heart is extremely electrical, more so than it's even a pump, so when you stop it, in theory, it restarts in a normal rhythm, rather than in the bad one you stopped.

So was I going to stop this sweet old lady's heart? I'd seen it done, and, as you can imagine, it doesn't feel good. When you shock someone in full arrest, running V tach, the heart can take minutes to restart, so you immediately continue CPR, and check the rhythm after a couple minutes. With SVT and A Fib, the heart only stops for a second or two. So they don't lose consciousness. But they kind of wish they had. If you have the time and balls, you sedate them first.

The benzo you use for this purpose, Versed, also erases the patient's memory of what happens, which is what cynics say is its real purpose. At least she doesn't remember. Though people's memory of pain is already pretty spotty. Or they wouldn't keep doing a lot of the shit that they keep doing.

By now I'm in the truck. I'm rolling. I'm going emergent even though the patient is stable. When in doubt....Better to go emergent by mistake than non emergent by mistake. I decide to call my ODS (on duty supervisor) Rick Slaughter for some advice.

"ODS. Slaughter."

I explain.

"Aw," he said, "Adenosine won't hurt her. But you ought to be transporting by now."

"We're in the truck."

Problem is, I don't have IV access. And can't get any. She has veins which would embarrass a spider. The spider would be hanging her thorax in shame, and the other spiders would be giggling. "Her mom couldn't weave worth shit either. It's amazing she survived." And even at that, her veins roll, shuck and jive.

So merrily we roll along. Nothing changes until we are pushing her stretcher into the ER. She remains alert and cheerful, her vitals are fine, she's warm pink and dry. Also still in SVT. 180 bpm.

It's hard to diagnose a really fast rhythm. 170 or 200 beats a minute is going to look regular, whether it's clockwork SVT, or irregularly irregular A Fib. What it can't be is a normal sinus tachycardia, because a person that age, unlike Lance Armstrong, can't run 170 normal beats a minute, much less 200.

This was SVT though. I had plenty of time to examine the strips in detail.

Well, as soon as we hit the door to the ER, her blood pressure drops to 70 systolic, she looks green and she wilts.

Had this happened in the truck, it would have been time to put on the pacing pads and shock. But we are in the ER by now so I'm going to wait for a consult. I haven't turned over care yet, so certainly if someone goes into pulseless V Tach, you would shock immediately wherever you are.

As we spot the doc in the offing, who has been alerted to a hot call coming in, her blood pressure drop and stress cardiovert my sweet old lady. So what the doc sees is a sweet old lady, bright and cheery, running a normal sinus rhythm on my monitor, with renewed perfectly stable vitals.

Well, she does still have the knots on her head. And she feels a little weak.

I'd smile sheepishly, but I do have the strips I have run to show him.

"Well," he says, "anyway she's running a perfectly normal rhythm now." He trots off. Got more important things to do right now than check out the lumps on her head.

The lesson here is that if you follow the protocols, then even if you have some lapses in experience or judgment, or even if you can't do what you would like to do, or can't even do what is called for, you can still get a good outcome. Because all the while I was deciding whether or not to give adenosine, whether or not to shock, when I was unable to get IV access, I was loading and transporting, monitoring and giving oxygen.

Ultimately, that's what we do. Transport to definitive care. Hand over to the guy making the big bucks.

In a very similar incident, we arrived to find a similar old lady, lying in bed, looking really sick this time. On the monitor, she really was in A Fib, RVR. Atrial fibrillation with rapid ventricular response. That is, her atrium was fibrillating uselessly and stimulating her ventricles to beat too fast to fill and pump enough blood.

Got her in the truck, got IV access this time, and decided I would shock. She did not have chest pain or shortness of breath, and her blood pressure was not really shocky either, which are the classical "symptomatic" markers of an A Fib RVR that you should shock and try to cardiovert, but she was so weak and sick that she could not even lift her head off the pillow. I considered that symptomatic. Her pressure was too low for the calcium channel blocker we carry to slow down a heart in RVR. Need 120 systolic, per protocol.

Now, you are cautious about shocking A Fib because you can dislodge clots that have formed in the fibrillating atrium, causing strokes and MI's. The hospital likes to put the patient on blood thinners for a while before cardioversion. Still, if a patient is symptomatic, as the phrase has it, you take the risk to fix the more immediate problem.

So I put the pads on her, set the joules to 100, which is the right dose for A Fib, as it is harder to cardiovert than SVT, and pushed the shock button. My poor patient yelps and goes completely unconscious. I am far from happy about this, but the monitor does show that after her heart stops for a couple seconds it resumes a nice normal sinus rhythm.

Then it goes right back into A Fib. A Fib is just really recalcitrant. I've never been able to cardiovert it. They do, sometimes, in hospitals, so it is possible, but even there they don't always succeed.

Pretty soon she does wake up, though, and says she feels better. I don't know why since she's back in the exact same rhythm. I got exactly two beats of normal sinus. Maybe she is being nice, or optimistic.

Her pressure is a little stronger, so I could administer the calcium channel blocker now, but it can drop blood pressure really badly, so I decide I've fucked with this poor lady enough. We're near Wilford Hall, anyway.

They administer the channel blocker. It works.

It may surprise you that a person can be too weak to lift her head and also be hypertensive. It did me at first too. But hypertension is a strange disease, practically ubiquitous in older people in our society. The silent killer. You don't realize you have it until you have a stroke or heart attack.

Like cardiac artery disease. In 30% of cases the first symptom is sudden death.

And who would imagine that if your heart is too weak to pump all the fluid out of your body, which is called congestive heart failure, you would also have hypertension, which is your heart pumping too strongly, as it were. But not only can you, it's the usual finding. In fact, HTN causes CHF.

So again, this could hardly be called a successful call. I diagnosed the problem correctly this time, and was able to administer the required intervention, as well as get IV access, but the intervention did not work. Causing me either to lose my nerve, or to take a more conservative approach, however you like to see it. Still and all, I also transported expeditiously, so the ER was able to recover the fumble.

The same can be said for another old lady, this one originating in an armed forces retirement community. It's quite a beautiful facility, officers only, so you get to meet fighter jockeys, men who jumped into Nijmegen, Generals and their wives. This time it was a very elegant couple indeed. Age 80, the Colonel was obviously still enamoured, an awed admirer of his wife, who I thought might be recent for that reason She was an elegant, understated but glamorous lady, also in her eighties, with beautifully polished nails finishing her aged and veiny hands.

She felt terrible, and her blood pressure was dangerously low. The reason it was low was her heart was only running at 32 beats a minute. Sinus brady. I attempted IV access on scene with the object of infusing a half mg of atropine, which usually works admirably for bradycardia. Fluid or possibly dopamine to follow, for the hypotension, if it didn't resolve.

Once again I was absolutely unable to gain IV access. I only made two attempts on scene, and then another in route, because the protocol, once again, is rapid transport after no more than two attempts.

She was hanging in there bravely and laconically when we got there, with an understated, sophisticated irony, a smile like Lauren Bacall's, and she was still hanging in there bravely by the time we got her to Big Willie.

So again the lesson is, the protocols are well designed. They are redundant, like the design of an airplane. If one thing doesn't work, or even if you do something wrong, or fail something you do attempt, the protocols will save your ass, to say nothing of the patient's. And no reasonable, well informed medical authority, looking over your shoulder after the fact, will fail to understand. They will know that an emergency is an unplanned event, and the response to it is never perfect and sometimes things go a whole lot less than perfect. And still turn out well most of the time, because of something else that you did do right.

And the remarkable resilience of the human body.

MOI

MOI stands for mode of injury. It can be quite useful. If a broken leg was caused by getting whacked on the leg by a hoof, you look for completely different things than if it's caused by a high speed MVA.

MOI can be useful if in a lot of ways. We were on a three man truck once--I was a field training recruit--and we had to respond all the way across town for a head injury. All the nearby trucks were tied up with other calls.

So it took more than 20 minutes to get there. It happens.

My field training officer's regular partner was in distress though. He had needed to pee even before we got in route and by the time we got to the scene he was bursting at the seams.

On scene he was understandably and visibly more occupied by his own physical problem than the patient's.

We found a cantankerous old Vietnam vet, drunk, in a wheelchair, with multiple medical problems, mostly brought on by his own doings, as well as what had happened to him in Nam. His admiring son in law was there--he had called us. He told us our patient was a hero. Silver star. Now, there are many more Vietnam vets than actually served, I mean many many more, and it sometimes seems all of them got medals, as well as PTSD, even the ones who never left their desk chair. But we thanked him politely and sincerely for his service all the same.

He had fallen and hit his head, which was bruised and bleeding. How did this happen? He slipped--in the bathroom, striking his forehead on the edge of the bathtub.

"Oh, ah," my partner said, raising his finger. "I'll go check out the MOI." And with that he headed to the bathroom. I mean, you can't just ask an injured person if you can use his bathroom the minute you get on an emergency scene. In fact, you try not to use their bathrooms at all.

But checking out the MOI, that was his clear duty.

Rick and I tended to the patient, and soon we heard aural evidence that our partner was being very thorough. He had clearly checked out the toilet flush device while he was in there examining the bathtub.

Always good to go the extra mile. Check out the patient's ADLs while you're there. Make sure he can eat, bathe, clean and clothe himself, the fridge is working, there is food available, the tub and toilet are in order. Make sure it can actually flush urine, not just swirl.

HOSPICE

Hospice care is basically a very good thing, when it is used appropriately, flexibly and sensitively. Statistics show that hospice patients who have been honestly judged to be in the last 6 months or so of their lives due to incurable diseases or conditions actually live longer, as well as more comfortably, than patients who continue to receive aggressive medical interventions. This is because the medical interventions for such patients are basically useless, surely cannot provide a cure or long term management, and tend to be uncomfortable and debilitating in their own right. Medical intervention is always a balancing of side effects against positive effects and down sides. No one would incur all the problems caused by blood thinners or chemo if they did not justifiably fear the consequence of not taking them--stroke or cancer--even more. In the terminally ill, the down side outweighs the benefit. Which is nil.

Furthermore, hospice saves everyone a lot of money. It is hard to balance life and health against money, but balancing negligible gains in longevity of very poor quality against aggressive but useless interventions means balancing negligible gains, or even just prolonged suffering, against a fortune, in many cases. Money and resources that then cannot be used for better purposes.

What this has come to mean, though, is that hospice care is very lucrative for providers. Medicare and other insurance providers are pleased to pay hospice organizations handsomely, since that means they will not have to pay for more expensive, if useless, attempts to prolong life. And this in turn means that some less than noble, in fact in some cases sleazy, operators have been attracted to these programs like vultures to carrion. Exactly like vultures to carrion.

I have observed over the years that hospice organizations that I much admired for their compassion and professionalism, for their soothing, luxurious accommodations for the terminally ill and their families, their sensitive handling of medical problems, have continued to prosper alongside an increasing number of more mediocre organizations. Even some of the worst nursing homes we visit are getting into the act with hospice wings which neglect patients in squalid conditions.

Studies show that for-profit providers, as opposed to non-profits, show patient data indicating that their patients stay on hospice longer, and not infrequently even LEAVE hospice, not through dying but through being discharged (cured!). That's because for-profits take on patients with less serious conditions. Why is simple. A for-profit organization is for profit. It is in their financial interest to keep patients longer, and take on patients who need less care. In theory, their ideal patient would be a healthy young person who required no care at all and could stay on hospice for decades. So there is a strong incentive to accept patients who are not really in the last 6 months of their lives, who can live at home instead of in the facility, and who don't require frequent or difficult home visits by nursing staff. (Hospice patients spend as much time at home as possible, but often have to come to facility beds, either for more involved care or because their families cannot be with them for 24 hours a day or cannot lift, clean or take care of them.) It is also in the for-profits' interest to provide less care, even to bully families who ask for more care, for example IV fluid rehydration. They tell families that those interventions would automatically take the patient off hospice, which is not true. A hospice patient can't be on a vent or pressors or chemotherapy--all of which would mean that aggressive or invasive means are still being employed, to cure the incurable— but measures which make the process of dying more comfortable, or gently prolong the life of patients who are not suffering, and who still have a quality of life that they consider worthwhile, surely are warranted.

In this particular instance, the free market does not stack up well against non-profits. Unfortunately, given how effective the free market can be, this is frequently the case with medical care. Patients don't really fit the ideal definition of consumers. And the outcome desired is not cheaper prices or bigger profits but better health care.

Even some of the better hospice organizations, though not the best ones, have started to bully patients and families in a way I will describe in the following stories.

Let's start with a good one, though, since hospice really is a good idea and is usually well executed.

Now, a good hospice story is a dubious proposition. It takes an optimistic, almost Pollyanna-like person to consider a story about someone dying to be a good read.

Still, a story where a patient gets what she wants and is treated not only considerately but brilliantly is a good hospice story.

We were met by family and nursing staff even before we made contact with this lady in her hospital bed. We often handle all this stuff by ourselves, but it's nice to get some info and assistance. The story was that she was only in her late 40's but had acute and total kidney failure. Plenty of hospice patients are young, even children. All it requires is a terminal condition. But most are old.

It's remarkable in the age of dialysis, but not long ago kidney failure was a death sentence, and in short order. Proust died of it in his 40's, earlier in the last century.

Now, among the eery venues medics inhabit, unlike ordinary citizens--one part of medics' parallel universe, among the crime scenes, traffic disasters, among the dead, sick and maimed, in our alternate reality, not in a different dimension but right here next to McDonald's--are dialysis centers. Zombie apocalypse. White, quiet, sterile, icy, enormous caverns, where antiseptic vampire machines visibly suck the blood out of 20 or more victims simultaneously, victims who are asleep, watching TV on little monitors, semi-comatose, missing limbs, gangrenous, bloated, or sometimes just healthy-looking, normal-appearing people. Some come in on stretchers, some drive up and walk in. Three times a week for four hours at a pop, they bare their dialysis site, the artificial shunt a surgeon has implanted between an artery and vein, where he judges by the "thrill" he can hear through a stethoscope whether it's working, and attendants stick needles into their prey and then the machines suck out every drop of their blood, clean it, and return it to their bodies, complete with additives like blood thinners to keep it all from coagulating into a yellow, reeking pudding. That's if all goes well.

If not, they call us. We run the full arrest behind a not so discreet screen. Perform our interventions to support blood pressure, or heart rate, and transport. ABCD. Airway, breathing, circulation, diesel.

By the way, speaking of watching TV under all conditions, did you know that it is illegal to lock up an American in a room with no TV? Yeah, it's right in the constitution. I forget which article. Amazing foresight, those founding fathers. Check out your local nursing home. You'll see.

In our time, though, the dialysis center, while discreet, is ubiquitous. I live in a small town, and it has three of them. Of course this is Texas, majority obese, majority poor diet, majority Hispanic.

And very lucrative engines of commerce they are. At $300 plus for the ambulance transport for a good percentage of the patients, that's 6 trips per week back and forth, well, that's not even the charge for the dialysis itself. Attendants, exorbitantly priced (as always) medical equipment, an RN on scene, a nephrologist on call. Transport is only the tip of the iceberg. Transport from, of course, Specialized Nursing Facilities, SNFs, called sniffs, aka nursing homes, or, euphemistically, rehab facilities. What do you imagine it costs to keep one dialysis patient alive for one year?

If you call that life. Now, I would, if it were me, depending on how sick I was, but my patient did not: to return to my hospice call.

Namely, her story was, we were informed, that she had refused dialysis. We were warned not to even mention the D word in her presence. She also, that is, had an anxiety disorder. And a number of relatives who had been on dialysis. Based on her observation of their lives, she was having none of it.

Again, an adult who can answer four questions correctly can refuse medical care. They are: what is your full name? Where are you? What is today's date, or at least the year and month? What was the first question? Or otherwise indicate you know what is going on, now. For instance the name of the President.

I always think it's unfair when the emergency department nurse asks my patients where they are. I mean, I brought them there, and, if it's emergent, without consulting them much. So they didn't ask to come there, often they weren't the ones to call us in the first place, and no one told them, among all the hullaballoo, where they were going. Unlike me and the nurse, they're not familiar with all the hospitals in town. So how the heck would they know where they are? The RN is taking unfair advantage of our experience. I mean, one of the answers the patients give is, "Nurse, don't you know where you are? If not, should you be taking care of me?" Then again, if you deprive me of my watch and cell phone, I won't know what the date or day of the week is either, half the time. So I'll ask patients what city they're in and what month or year it is.

"Do you know what year it is?"

"Yes."

"Well, could you tell me?"

They get offended. Especially when they're sure it's 1987. Or if they don't want to admit they don't know.

So the family and nurse met us at her door to get us oriented. Do not, we were told, under any circumstances, say the D word. Dialysis.

So we walked into her hospital room, leaving the stretcher discreetly behind for the time being. She looked pretty good. Sick and anxious but basically reasonably healthy. Good color, alert, all her limbs intact, warm, pink and dry, good tone etc. The only thing at all remarkable in the room was the oxygen regulator, which was blowing oxygen out the Christmas tree into her nonrebreather mask at 25 liters a minute.

No human being needs 25 liters of O2. Elephants with severe COPD or CHF exacerbation don't need 25 liters O2. Maybe blue whales with pneumonia.

If the bag on the nonrebreather mask is full, more O2 just spills into the environment. We were getting lightheaded just being near her. I've seen big guys gasping for air suck down 15 liters, but even that is rare, and usually hyperventilation.

I turned it down, looking at the NRB bag to make sure it stayed full. She started screaming. I turned it back up. I think the hissing white noise was calming her down.

Other than that giant sucking or hissing sound, transport was uneventful. She did not want to talk and anyway couldn't with a NRB over her face whooshing O2 over the bedsheets. We barely made it to the truck, though, before the D tank was dry.

The M tank on the truck is huge and the transport was short, less than a mile, but even so she sucked it dry. I did try to turn it down again, but only once. I'd rather hear whooshing O2 draining my oxygen supply than women screaming. Being a little lightheaded was a small price to pay for intact hearing.

I was wondering how Vitas Hospice was going to handle this. It's one of the good ones, the best in my opinion. Very concerned, adroit, competent staff; beautiful, quiet, soothing rooms. I was ready to move in. But they only have O2 converters capable of delivering 6 liters. Any problems, they either let the patient succumb or they call us.

The RN, a person I admire for wisdom and medical expertise (she worked in an ICU before tapering off), took one look at my patient, drew up a syringe of morphine, and decanted it into a vein.

Fixed.

I was impressed. Patient resting comfortably on 2 liters O2 via nasal cannula. Hospices give morphine for everything. Anxiety, shortness of breath, sciatica, eczema. If you don't have to worry about addiction, constipation, or side effects, it's a perfect drug. Patient feels great, cures anxiety; she sleeps well, no pain. It actually helps breathing, edema and heart function.

We give it for severe pain, for cardiac chest pain and congestive heart failure. I had never seen it used for anxiety. Valium would not have done for this patient really as it can depress respiration. It would have been an option, since she was not really in any respiratory difficulties, but we tend to hoard it for seizures or sedation. A couple mg wouldn't have touched her.

"Wow," I said to the nurse. "That solved a nasty problem."

"Rough transport?"

"Yeah. I could probably use some morphine if you have any left."

She just smiled. You're not allowed to laugh out loud at Hospice.

Just to give you an idea of the follow up consequences of any call, which never exists in isolation—the calls keep coming till you're off shift—we got a call for respiratory distress next. I declined it. I had half a little D tank left. The main was drained.

Dispatcher was freaked out and pissed. Even after I explained the problem he said the patient probably wouldn't need more than I had.

This is true. Most respiratory distress calls are handled adequately with a nasal cannula running a couple liters. Still, can't take the risk. A genuine respiratory failure, or severe problem, with an NRB or c pap running at 10 liters, can drain a D tank in less time than it takes to get to a hospital. An ambulance with no oxygen is a diesel RV.

"You can send a BLS truck for back-up, or to first respond, and I can use their oxygen, but I can't take a respiratory distress with no O2."

So he sent me all the way across town, running code, for an Altered Mental Status r/o sepsis instead.

"And what makes you sure an AMS patient won't need oxygen?" I said.

"He won't. Just take the call."

"Yeah, you wuss, take the call," the medic who had been redirected to take my respiratory distress jumped in on the radio to say. On the radio. I could understand he was pissed but I was stunned and enraged by the lack of professionalism. What he said was really pushing it just between the two of us, and totally unacceptable for radio traffic. This new service was a lot more rough and ready than I considered to be good practice. In time I found they were not averse to running hot just to improve their response times to non-emergent calls.

So I wrote both of them up on report afterwards, only the second time I'd ever done that in 7 years (I believe in watching my colleague's backs).

I did run the call. We got stuck in construction and had another unpleasant moment on the radio when I explained we would be delayed. Another dispatcher took over to calm things down.

Got to the nursing home and discovered why I had run hot all the way across town, and why the dispatcher had known I wouldn't need much oxygen.

The RN who received us was a willowy, dark haired, pleasant and calm young woman who first asked us why she had been getting updates from the second dispatcher about our ETA. "They never did that before on calls." Calm, homey and efficient nursing home. Luxurious in a down to earth way, not professionally decorated. Military. Lot of wood and stuffed chairs, fireplaces and birds. An old dog.

"You didn't tell the first dispatcher it was an emergency?"

"No." She made it two syllables, a doubting tone.

"It's not a septic wound infection?"

"Well, it's infected, but he isn't septic. Just has to go sometime today."

"Well, is he altered mental? Or didn't you say that either?

"Sure he's altered, he's got dementia, but it's no worse than usual. Not really ALTERED."

So that's why the dispatcher had known I wouldn't need a lot of oxygen. And he had run me code all the way across town mostly because the call came after my deactivation time, when I can refuse non-emergency calls, which he figured I would, given the lack of oxygen and warm fellowship.

And that's why he got writ up. Being unprofessional on the radio is bad enough, but sending an ambulance lights and sirens across town for a call he knows is not emergent is illegal, not to put too fine a point on it. You don't risk crews and passersby, disrupt traffic and abuse the public's patience for a non-emergent call, even given that code calls are run relatively safely.

So that was the "good" hospice call. Of course there were many more, too uneventful to stick in the mind. Carting dying people, half dead people. Not exactly saving lives. Took some getting used to. Medicine encompasses many things, including helping people die.

So here's one of the bad ones. It emphasized an unpleasant fact about transport calls vs emergency response. In a 911 call I can reasonably expect to save a patient, or at least improve his condition. People call me for an acute condition which I can often do something about. I can hope to check the box on my run form which indicates the patient's condition improved en route, rather than the ones which indicate his condition remained the same, or deteriorated. But when I transport someone--who is already sick enough to require ambulance transport--to his dialysis or doctor's appointment, or even to the emergency room because he got worse, often the best I can hope for, especially in the non-emergency room transports, is to get the patient to his destination in about the same condition I found him in. My function is to keep a patient with chronic disease stable, rather than to fix or ameliorate an acute problem. Discouraging. In a way, the guy can only go down. The best I can work for is no change. They can get worse or crash, otherwise they wouldn't need ambulance transport, but, particularly for hospice patients, I'm not hoping for improvement.

So we get called to an ICU to transport a patient home for hospice care. They have given up.

Worse, she's in such a bad state that they are not really sure she will make it. They have tried to take her off pressors, but her blood pressure keeps crashing. So I'm going to take her on a dopamine drip.

"Well, is she hospice or not? Does she have a DNR?" I ask. Hospice means no invasive procedures, no resuscitation, no intubation, no chemo and NO PRESSORS.

"Yeah, she does have a DNR, but she doesn't truly go on hospice until she gets home."

"So if she crashes in route I attempt to resuscitate?"

"Well, no, but she does stay on dopamine till you get there."

Well, I can't very well complain about hospices not being flexible enough if I'm not willing to go along when they ARE being flexible, so OK. Not totally happy about the legal situation, but I'm not a lawyer, so following MD instructions should serve.

In route we develop some problems with the IV pump occluding, getting air in the line, and sure enough she does start going hypotensive, but that's easily fixed.

It's a long trip. We're underway for two hours. In my initial assessment, I saw that she looked terrible. Which was fine. You want a hospice patient to be circling the drain. Doomed healthy-looking people are not right. But I find out that although she's so weak she can't lift her head, and can't speak above a whisper, she's not semi-comatose at all, not even confused or altered mental. She is in fact not only alert and oriented but articulate and intelligent. Not to my mind ready to die, other than physically. This is not increasing my comfort level with this call. You like your dying people to act like they're dying. Be beyond pain or fear.

Well, at least she is not in any pain, other than by being so weak. Still, if she's not in pain, and still alert, why are we giving up on prolonging life? Not my decision to make.

We finally get to a little run down house in a bare yard. It's hot, even at midnight. There are five or six relatives there. The dopamine in the 10 cc syringe in my pump is about to run out. I consider drawing up more from the dopamine bag I took along, from where I drew up the original syringe full, but she's supposed to go off dopamine at home. I take the bag in with me so I can do it inside if necessary. Dopamine is very powerful. It's measured in micrograms instead of milligrams, which is why even after a long trip the 10 cc syringe is still not empty.

We get our patient into her bed in a front room without incident. This time there is an actual hospice nurse, an RN at that, on scene. Often you run into all kinds of problems because the hospice has not adequately prepared the scene or told you what you need to know, and is nowhere to be found to boot. There's no oxygen, or the room is inaccessible by stretcher, and the patient too heavy to carry with two people. You have to call the local fire department. They're nice and take it in stride (they're firemen), but the family is not and doesn't.

The RN is a bear shaped young guy who looks fairly bright. One of those fashionable four day beards. Khaki pants, t shirt. Hasn't slept for a while. Shiny face. It's hot. Texas.

But now the problem is that Uncle Jaime is still in route, may not arrive for a couple hours, and the family, patient and Uncle Jaime himself all want him to say goodbye.

Medically, there is no reason this patient can't stay on a dopamine drip for another couple hours: for all I know, days. We, however, are not going to stay there with her, obviously. We provide transport. Hospice provides care. But the hospice nurse has no IV pump. Nor, normally, should he. Hospice patients are not supposed to be on a medical drip. Equally obviously, they can't keep our pump. Where I goeth, pump goeth.

It soon becomes clear that the RN has no intention of finding a pump somewhere and getting it here. Admittedly this would be a tall order. Convenience stores don't sell IV pumps; they're very expensive, like all medical equipment, and hospitals don't loan theirs out. I do point out that, even without the pump, the RN could depress the syringe a little every few minutes, and keep the dopamine going by hand. Would probably work. Certainly, if the pump broke down, and it was my task to keep the patient alive, that's what I would try.

Suggestion not appreciated.

RN looks harried. Hospice is supposed to be easy nursing. Give patient morphine, hold family's hand. Can't sell him our pump either, even if he were authorized to buy it.

I have some more suggestions, along the line of, why not keep the patient, who is not suffering, and who is fully alert and conscious, alive until she can complete her goodbyes, at least. But I don't say anything. People tell me, however, that I don't control my body language very well. Partly it's because I don't examine other people's body language closely most of the time, and am in fact not overly concerned with what they feel, as opposed to doing my job right, so I imagine they feel the same about me. This is an error along the lines of a toddler thinking that things that are out of sight, don't exist, or "If I don't see you, you can't see me'. It's called peek-a-boo, or, in an adult like me, magical thinking.

The RN is not looking at me anyway. Unlike Ronald Reagan, I have not made a friend. In fact, he's not looking at anyone, except if he can't help it, like at the patient's sister, who is addressing him.

So he kind of edges me out of the way, and tells her that she can revoke hospice, and then we, the ambulance, can take her sister to the emergency room; or....He doesn't know quite how to phrase it. Or she can let her croak. As prescribed.

He takes a breath and starts on a new tack. "Did you want to revoke hospice? Is that what your sister would like to do? We can do that at any time. I thought you had decided...."

No, no. They want hospice. She is dying. She is incurable, with a very short time to live no matter what steps are taken, and they want her to die comfortably, at home.

But they also would like her to die after Uncle Jaime, and, it turns out, Aunt Esther, and someone else, can get there.

Well, here's your consequence for taking a hospice patient home on a pressor drip, of being neither fish nor fowl.

You might begin to wonder, too, what's taking Uncle Jaime so long, given I have been en route for a couple hours, and even before that a decision was made to send this patient home on hospice. You would wonder this because you are an amateur. We professionals have long since stopped expecting rational behavior from our patients or their families. Mostly, they wouldn't even be our patients if they had exercised common sense.

On a 911 service, you are concerned about only one thing, the welfare of the patient, and the desires of the patient. On a transport service, however, you are at the mercy, to some extent, of the facility which called you, in this case hospice. Paramedics have a slogan they learn, 'treat the patient, not the monitor.' That is, if your cardiac monitor is showing some horrible, lethal rhythm you ought to shock, but you look up to find the patient is sitting up, talking to you, and appearing to be in no apparent distress, as the phrase has it, then you address the patient, keeping only your left eye on the monitor. As it were. Hoping it will shut the fuck up, act respectable and start doing its job right.

In a transport service, however, the rule tends to be, 'treat the facility, not the patient.' If the facility is happy, they will call you to transport the next patient. If not, not. Unlike with 911, the patient or family is rarely the person who calls you. Besides, with 911, if the patient or family are unhappy with your care, they can't call another 911. They can complain, and your director will look into it. He does tend to be on the side of his medics, people he knows and trusts, and has hired and promoted. An EMS director will be at the mid or end of long career in EMS. Not only is he knowledgeable and experienced, but well connected. He knows the mayor and the sheriff. Not easy to intimidate. If he decides his medics did the right thing, he's perfectly willing to tell the complainant to fuck off. Probably more politely than that, but, if necessary, to remind the complainant that interfering with a public servant in his duties is a felony, and he hopes it won't happen again.

The CEO of a transport service is in a different position. She wants the facility to call her rather than her competitor. She has built her business on facilities calling her. She doesn't really care whose fault the issue is. She wants the facility happy.

So, maybe too late, I was keeping my mouth shut. Though I may have had my shoulders sagging in despair and my mouth hanging open in disbelief, if my partner's comic imitation of my body language is at all accurate.

The RN took the family into the living room for further discussion. Or further bullying, however you want to see it.

The upshot was, the DNR/hospice remained in force, and the pump had to come off, Uncle Jaime or no Uncle Jaime.

Now, it was my pump. As far as the RN was concerned, it could stay there forever. So the onus was kind of on me to DC it. Namely, kill the patient.

"Do you want me to DC the pump?" I said. I was trying to catch his eye to show him I was fully cognizant of his strategy of edging me into the line of fire, otherwise under the bus, but he was not catching my eye.

"Yes," he said, looking the other way. Too busy, you know. Just standing there. I looked around at the family, but naturally they had no suggestions to make.

I DCed the pump. Legally, it might have made some kind of difference, but morally I couldn't see any difference between him doing it and me doing it. End result the same; decision making process the same. And not my call to make. I had transferred care and the RN outranked me.

Besides, I'm a paramedic. I do stuff. I don't just stand there and watch other people do stuff.

Then I hustled us out of there. It was late, we were tired, we wanted to go home. And also I estimated the patient would last only minutes off dopamine, and I preferred not to be there when she died. Particularly not if the family changed their mind, though that didn't seem likely.

So, Uncle Jaime, that's how it went down.

By now, it should be obvious what my feelings about this call were. What I like to do is save lives. That's kind of my job description, in my mind, even if most of the time it's just keeping patients in the same state they already are, or helping them in other ways. Still, helping them die, while it could be a noble thing, isn't exactly my thing.

I mean, by the same token, I'm not opposed to capital punishment, if it's reserved for rare, truly heinous crimes, and for perpetrators who we can be 100% sure did them. But I'm not going to start the IV or inject the lethal drugs. Against my oath.

The next day I told my supervisor about the call.

I said, "I used to save lives; now I kill people."

"You don't really think that, do you?" she said.

"Well, kind of. Not really, I guess."

Ok, one more bad hospice story. This one is not about bullying though.

It does happen though. My own mother was on hospice, and when I asked the social worker who was admitting us, how they felt about IV relief of dehydration, for example, if Mom needed it, she said, "Oh no, but we would give morphine, if, say, she were short of breath." So here was a social worker telling me, a paramedic, and my mother, a fully alert MD, how they would treat her SOB or hypotension, despite our wishes. We were not talking about a surgery or mechanical ventilation or intubation or anything.

I fired her. She said our independent living facility only used her hospice.

"So if I call security, I can't count on them to remove you? I gotta do it myself?"

"Morphine is, too, good for shortness of breath," she said, hurrying out in huff. Neither of us seemed to be in the mood for my comprehensive lecture on SOB.

No, this next patient was another story entirely. An obese, middle aged male we again picked up in an ICU, and who again was being transported a long way, from his little town's hospital to a hospice in San Antonio, a good hour or more away. And he was semi-comatose this time. GCS about 8. Withdrawing from pain, some muttering once in a while, no eye opening.

Once again, I was not convinced he would make it. I have an instinct for these things. Comes with the job. At least this time the DNR and hospice were all in order, though.

Except he was on a Bi-Pap. To explain, we use a CPAP, a continuous positive air pressure machine, to help a patient who cannot get enough air into his lungs because of sleep apnea or asthma or COPD. Bi-Pap, which adjusts the positive pressure, depending on whether the patient is exhaling or inhaling (less pressure for the exhale), is for chronic lung problems, like maybe severe cases of the above, or pulmonary fibrosis or the like.

For a while, though, we were finding hospice patients on Bi-Pap, though now the fashion seems to have changed again. What happened was, family members saw a dying patient laboring and gasping for breath, and wished something more could be done to make them comfortable, which is the goal of hospice, after all. Intubation and putting the patient on mechanical ventilation was not really an option. Then the patient would not be on hospice, but rather in an ICU or LTAC, long term acute care. Monitored and assisted even if he descended into a vegetative state.

So the legal alternative was Bi-Pap. It could help him breathe, but, being non-invasive, allow him to stay on hospice or palliative care. However, I think it's been going out of fashion again, because, first, in effect it can just be a vent without intubation. The mask fits tightly over his face, and the Bi-Pap can even be set to actually give breaths, not just positive pressure. Second, the patient may seem to be suffering less in the short term, but the net effect is just to prolong the agony of the dying process. To die, you're going to have to stop breathing, and then (or instead), your heart has to stop. Keeping the person breathing beyond what he can do himself prolongs this process, indefinitely. Until he becomes vegetative, or until he is cured, if he has a curable condition. That's not hospice though. Hospice is when you shift to keeping the patient comfortable, from trying to cure him. Even though, paradoxically, he probably will live longer on hospice, if his condition is terminal, than if you keep stressing him with useless interventions.

So we trundled our hospice patient out of the ICU to our ambulance. He stank, he was slick with sweat and pale of skin. When you can't breathe, or are dying, you go onto shock.

This was all quite satisfying. We want our dying hospice patient to appear to be dying. We don't like to withhold interventions from a healthy looking, alert patient, even when a doctor tells us he doesn't have long to live. We don't disagree, but it's just sad.

What was not satisfying was my sense that we were not going to deliver him to the hospice alive. In confirmation, even before we got out the hospital door, his oxygen SAT had dropped from 100 or 99 % to 92. 92 isn't that bad. Anything over 95 is great, over 90 is OK, and in COPD patients, even 88 can be tolerated by some. But I didn't like him dropping 8 points like that.

Well, he held that SAT pretty well for a while, but then he dropped into the upper 80s, then 70s. Not good. On 100% oxygen already. He was not going to be able to maintain that. I couldn't give him more than 100% O2, and of course breathing for him via intubation or a bag valve mask was out. DNR. Do not resuscitate. Do not intubate, do not bag, no pressors. No cardiac drugs.

The Bi-Pap seemed to be doing a lot of work too. I wasn't seeing him breathing on his own much at all. I called ahead to the hospice unit to warn them. If he died, I would still bring him there.

Plus his heart rate was not going up. Anyone who can't breathe or whose SATs drop is going to become tachycardic, unless he is on medication (say for hypertension or arrhythmias) which holds his heart rate down. This guy, though, per hospice protocol, had been taken off all his meds. Which was why he was going downhill so fast. So that meant that his heart rate not going up was really ominous. It was in effect relative bradycardia, judged by his condition, rather than the absolute definition of 60 to 100 beats per minute.

So I decided to stick him on a cardiac monitor. DNR and hospice patients aren't really supposed to be on a monitor, since you are not going to do anything about what you find anyway, but I wasn't proposing to record an EKG, or document it, or do anything based on what I found. I just wanted to know what was going on.

So he's running a nice, even rhythm. *With pacer spikes.* I had taken his history, meds (none anymore) and demographics with me for my run form, but no one had mentioned anything about a pacemaker. With a hospice patient, you're supposed to turn off the pacemaker, and especially the internal defibrillator. If you're not allowed to externally pace or defibrillate a patient, due to his hospice status, what sense does it make to have an internal pacemaker doing the same thing?

So the Bi-Pap was breathing for him, and the pacemaker was keeping his heart beating. Essentially he was dead, and I was running my own little moving ICU, keeping him in a vegetative state. All I needed was dopamine.

Well, even a pacemaker can only do so much, so by the time I got to the hospice, he was running only pacemaker spikes, with the occasional agonal beat in response.

When we unloaded him, his family was right there, and also the hospice nurse, who had come outside, alerted by my phone call. She asked me if he was dead. I discreetly cut my fingers across my throat to indicate he was finished, without alarming the family, who were of course hoping for at least a few minutes in the nice, quiet, luxury hotel atmosphere of the hospice room, as opposed to seeing Dad dead in the parking lot.

"What?" the nurse said in a loud voice. "Is he...?"

"Yeah," I muttered, frowning at her.

So we took him inside, pacemaker and Bi-Pap cheerfully doing their jobs. We put him on the bed, with the nurse asking the family to wait outside until we got him settled.

She put a stethoscope on his chest to pronounce, a fairly useless ritual. Stethoscopes are great, but heart tones and breathing are hard to hear if they're very reduced.

"I can put the monitor on him," I said.

"OK. Please."

Meanwhile she had taken him off the Bi-Pap so he wasn't breathing any more.

Well, the monitor showed some heart rhythm, actually. So she put him back on the Bi-Pap.

"It's really only agonal," I said. I mean, we were trying to let him go, not prolong things.

"Agonal, yeah."

She took him back off.

I trooped out about the time the family trooped in. Once again, I had to check the "worse" box for whether the patient's condition had improved, stayed the same or worsened during transport. Fortunately I didn't have to explain why, it was obvious with a hospice patient, but still, I like to check "improved."

On 911 calls, I mostly could.

GRIM REAPER AMBULANCE SERVICE

Every time I get tired of problems at work, I can imagine starting my own ambulance company.

All you need is a TDH approved and equipped ambulance, a partner, and one or two patients. I mean, think about it. A transport costs 300$, plus $35 a mile. $400, even. Every dialysis patient needs a round trip three times a week. That's more than 1200 bucks. If you could get two of them referred to you, you and your partner would make 1200 a week each. 50K a year after expenses, for maybe two hours a day, three days a week. Imagine you had 6 or 7 patients. Now you know why you see so many ambulance companies, "mom and pops" as they are called.

We had a guy we took every week, 3 times a week, who still lived independently at home. He got around via motorized wheelchair. House was dirty but he and his also handicapped wife seemed to manage.

"You know," I said once, "you could go by wheelchair van or even taxi, actually."

"A taxi costs 30 bucks a pop," he said. "I couldn't afford that three times a week."

"But an ambulance is more than 300."

"Yeah, but insurance pays for that." Anyone on dialysis automatically gets Medicare, though some drive themselves. And Medicare still beats private insurance coverage all silly.

Medicare does not pay for wheelchair vans. I don't know why. Cost is hardly more than a taxi.

I could take him in my car, throw in coffee and cookies, and make more than I do working four 12 hour shifts all week, but insurance wouldn't pay for my car either.

My company would be called Grim Reaper Ambulance. We would paint the truck black, with red trim, and stencil on our motto. "Everybody's gotta go sometime."

For some reason my boss doesn't feel threatened.

Point being, there are huge savings available all across the board in health care, without compromising patient care in the least. As another example, if you made it easy for a nursing home medical director to admit patients directly to hospital beds, say for a confirmed broken hip or CHF follow up, they would not be sending them there via emergency rooms, tying ERs up with unnecessary patients and costing thousands of dollars for redundant work ups. Some docs do admit directly, but it's a lot to ask of a busy MD, the hours of unpaid hassle dealing with insurance and hospital admission clerks. That's what we get paid for. Handsomely, at least the owners.

MY HERO: PEOPLE I ADMIRE

Well, there's Martin Luther King...no, this is a book about EMS. There have been many really good medics I have known, cool competent people like Bruce Richie, Ron Butcher, Pete Roth. Those are undisguised real names, unlike the others in my stories. But instead let me tell you about someone even more inspirational, working from even more difficult circumstances.

We were sitting in the truck outside a nursing home after dropping off a patient. I was feeling disgruntled owing to having to run back to back BLS calls for days, weeks, it seemed like years. My partner thought she was a salesperson rather than a medic: that is, she got along great with staff and was super polite and tactful. But, driving, she didn't seem to understand the difference between North and South, nor, medically, between a patient who was temporarily altered but baseline normal, and one who was permanently out to lunch, not home anymore: between sepsis and Alzheimer's. And this was pissing me off more than it normally would. I was hungry. Tired. Old and grouchy.

I was reading the paper, actually, taking a five minute break. My partner was nervously offering to drive, if I wanted to read the paper.

"I don't want to read, I want a break," I growled. "Randy always takes a full half hour at destination, smoke break and all."

"Randy got fired."

"Yeah, but not for that."

And just at this moment we got a really inspirational call. Pollyanna was looking out for us. Particularly for my anxious partner. Stuck between her medic and her boss.

At first I didn't even want to respond to it, until I was damn good and ready: had finished my run form and cleared. Yeah, it was another so called emergency, but this particular dispatcher had been sending us emergent to Altered Mental Status calls where the patient had been altered mental for days, and whose baseline was severe dementia to start with. He'd sent us half way across town during rush hour, lights and sirens, for a cantankerous old Vietnam vet who had stubbed his toe. Besides which, the guy didn't want to go to the hospital, with good reason, and had told his nursing staff that in the same no uncertain and unprintable terms with which he told us. He did offer to go if we gave him a pint of vodka, but we aren't allowed to carry that in the truck, useful as it might be.

But then I looked at the pager, which had gone off just about simultaneously with the radio call. We were going to another nursing home to pick up a staff member who was covered with fire extinguisher powder. She had been sprayed by a resident.

"Well, this I gotta see," I said.

"32, page received, in route," I said into the mike, once I keyed it up.

I lit it up. The nursing home we were responding to was the one where there are three EMS usable entrances, and one front entrance we are not allowed to use, and where you can never get anyone's attention at any of the EMS ones, because it's always the wrong one. But this time, since it wasn't a question of a possibly dying patient, but rather of them needing our help with a patient giving staff a hard time, they gladly opened the door we chose.

The scene inside was everything I could have hoped for. And it got better.

There was an angry old dude backed into a corner, holding off several nurses and staff people with a fire extinguisher he had wrestled from the wall, with remarkable ingenuity and resourcefulness. Especially considering he was in the Alzheimer's unit.

See, it proves Ronald Reagan could, too, be a great President, even when he was slipping a bit! He had a hands-off management style to start with. An inspiration to us all. Especially those of us getting along in years, subject to the odd senior moment. "I don't believe my opponent's youth and inexperience should be made an issue in this election," as Reagan himself said. Witty guy. Sense of humor intact until the end.

The staff consensus was that we, the ambulance crew, should rush the dude and subdue him. We were the paramilitary heroes, after all. But the only argument I saw in favor of that solution was the undoubted fact that fire extinguisher powder is completely harmless. My own consensus was that we should take tactical and strategic advantage of the limited resources of our opponent. At 87 years old, the guy was certainly going to tire, if he had not already. Merely standing up was a stretch for him. I could take one look and see he was on his last legs. Then, too, observing the amount of powder, it was clear to cooler and more experienced heads, like mine, that he was about out of ammo. Our second crew came in about then. We were, after all, going to have two patients. Our floured and breaded nurse, looking like a chicken ready for the deep fryer, and our hero.

I got the staff to clear the scene—they had had enough of it anyway—and sidled up closer to the terrorist, cautiously, keeping out of range. "Hey buddy," I said. "I see they haven't been treating you right here. Is that right?"

"Damn straight," he said, visibly relaxing a bit. Clearly an acute strategist as well as tactician, he had recognized he sorely needed reinforcements, and here they were. This was one of the few times I was grateful for my boss's otherwise unfortunate choice of navy blue for our uniforms. Most of the time, the last thing you want to be is an unarmed policeman. Besides, I hate navy blue. Let black be black, and let blue stay in Holland.

"Well, let's get you out of here and find you a better place to live. We can help you file a complaint." This was a win/win, as staff surely didn't want him back after he got discharged from the ER.

Meanwhile, of course, I had been assessing him. He looked confused, and tired. Bit of Alzheimer stiffness in the face. Bent a little, either bad back or kyphosis, osteoporosis. He was breathing well and talking sensibly, he was standing up on his own two feet, good muscle tone, his color was not bad, he wasn't panting more than could be expected, given his heroic efforts. He was focusing his eyes clearly on me. He did have a good sized skin tear on his right, extinguisher-bearing, arm from the struggle. That assessment would do handily until we could get some vitals and a history.

Meanwhile, my back up Basic crew was responding admirably. They had kept out of sight and well back to avoid giving the appearance of being threatening. Being a couple of experienced firefighters, they had reassured the nurse that she had every chance of living a long and pleasant life.

My own partner was standing around with her finger up her ass, clueless as usual. A lost sheep. There is always something to be done on an emergency scene. Collect data, take blood pressure, get stretcher ready. If you are doing nothing, you are doing it wrong.

I do have to say in her defense that I too once believed EMS was a spectator sport: when I was a newbie, watching my paramedic work. It somehow hadn't dawned on me yet that all the things they had taught me to do in school, with all that equipment, was not just for passing exams. I was actually expected to do that stuff on real people in real life.

The two firemen now eased their stretcher closer, seeing how things were going, and we settled my new buddy on it, and I handed over care after a brief check.

Then I turned my attention to patient number two, who turned out to be almost equally delightful. Normally, we take care of our own first. Had there been an injured firefighter or medic or cop, even if less injured than others, I would have seen to him before my terrorist. Staff in nursing homes should count, but....well....Besides, the old dude was in crisis, and the LVN merely breaded.

Anyway, once over the first shock, and reassured about extinguisher powder, she was taking it in good spirit. Working in a nursing home must be pretty deadly, even if you are in good one which isn't understaffed and reeking of puddles of urinary tract infection, so here was some excitement and entertainment.

She was a roly poly, bouncy haired, cheerful black lady with, it turned out, a good sense of humor. Glowing skin, big smile. Kind of a reverse Al Jolson, in white face instead of black face. Like a toddler who had applied the wrong color of Mommy's pancake make-up.

It was hard to imagine her abusing or terrorizing my old buddy, but the story is, we are not necessarily talking about abuse in the sense that people hit him, or denied care, or neglected him, or failed to see that he and his room were clean, as this was a pretty decent place. But the fact is that even a decent nursing home is pretty similar to a prison. Staff tell the inmates what they're going to eat, when they go to bed, when they are going to the doctor. They can't leave. Even staff who are not mean can easily be condescending or impatient or patronizing or dismissive.

In her case, I figured, either she had another side to her, or she had got exasperated with him, or she had somehow got into the crossfire, an innocent victim. I was not willing to entertain any bad thoughts about my hero having perhaps overreacted to gentle care with demented rage. I was on his side. I've seen too many abused elders.

Bonnie was perfectly OK with us taking her to the ER. The protocol was, any staff member who was injured was required to be checked out in the local ER. All she really needed was a bath and a change of clothes, but a trip to the ER might beat returning to work. She made sure to snag her lunch first, and then settled herself agreeably on the stretcher.

"Why not get someone to take her there by car, rather than via a 300$+ ambulance trip?" you ask. Well might you ask that question, since you are the one paying for it. Either through your taxes or your health insurance premiums. But, as for us medics, ours is not to reason why, ours is but to do or--well, we're not likely to die, actually, just collect our pay check. You call, we haul.

"Should I take you to the Methodist ER, or the deep fryer at Chicken Express?" I asked. It was pointless to even try dusting her off. White floury powder was coating her eyebrows, hair, clothes, shoes. Had she had pink instead of dark skin peeping through she might have looked like Santa Claus.

"If I get a choice, Chicken Express," she said. "I could use some fried chicken. Or how about the Thai place near 35?"

"Yeah, I think we could all use a margarita. But first, though, are you sure the nursing home is paying for this? My service charges employees who get transported by our ambulances, even with on the job injuries, I think." I mentioned this because I was taken with her and didn't want to repay her cheerful companionship with a nasty unexpected medical bill. Rather than being mad at our old buddy, or being sanctimonious, she was taking his shenanigans in the same spirit we were.

She shot up off the stretcher like it was on fire, forgetting she was covered head to toe with fire retardant.

"I'm for sure not going anywhere if I have to pay." She was under no professional illusions about ambulance transport costs.

So we waited around for a bit, while she trotted off to consult with her boss, the director of nursing. Our old terrorist buddy was long in route by the time she came back and settled herself back on our stretcher.

"Yeah, they're paying. Let's rock and roll!"

"Dja get it in writing?"

We had a jolly time en route. I declined to start an IV or do anything other than taking her vitals. I had fun explaining to the ER why we were coming in. Chief complaint, fire retardant OD. "But that stuff is harmless."

"Hey, you're talking to a fireman."

"No injuries? Stable vitals? WHY is she coming in?"

"No. Yes. Honestly, she got sprayed by a fire extinguisher, and the nursing home is insisting she get medical clearance before going back work. She's NAD." Which means no apparent distress.

"Oh all right then," the RN said in a resigned voice. She was not amused. RNs have real stuff to do, not just be farting around acting childish like us medics.

We never saw Ben, our elderly terrorist, again, other than briefly at the ER when we came in. The Basics told me transport was uneventful, which means they had continued to treat him with respect and tact in route. Plus he was pretty tired. I hope he found himself a better home, but I doubt it. The nursing home we took him from wasn't the best but it was better than average. Not unlikely, the ER had to discharge him to a worse one. So, not just a hero, but a tragic hero. Under the meaning of the act. Minotaur mazes, Augean stables, fiery furnaces, lion dens, pschah! Who wouldn't prefer any of them to a bad nursing home?

So he's still my hero. I'm taking it that staff in the nursing home were forcing him to do something he didn't want to do—official oppression—or treating him disrespectfully. I can't prove it, but even if we don't give him the benefit of the doubt--and to me he's more than innocent till proven guilty—then shit happens at enough nursing homes so he can be a symbol for all of their patients, the way we pick one particular soldier or civil rights worker, who may not even have been the best example to pick, and let her stand for all the things we admire in that field.

A personal disclosure here: I think everyone dies too soon. And declines too fast. My dad died when he was 65 of cardiac disease; my mom when she was 93, of breast cancer. With him, people will say, "Aw, that's young"; with her, they'll say what she herself said, "I had a good life," that is, a long life. No, in my opinion. They both died too young. I miss them.

I miss Fats Waller. I don't know how old he was when he died, and I do know he must have been born well before 1920, so he would hardly be around anymore, no matter how long-lived. But think how many rent parties he could still play. What a wonderful pianist. What a wit. That grin. Those hands.

He's easier to talk about than my Dad and Mom. But, naturally, I miss them even more. I think death is unfair. Unjust. My professional struggle with it is ultimately a failure. And personally, I don't want to live a good long life, I would rather be around when my kids have kids. I want to see them grow up too. I want to see what tech apps and what medical care we have in the 22nd century. The only positive thing I can see about dying is, I won't have to learn to use any more apps and electronic inventions. User friendly, my ass.

Now, when I was I high school, I admired a poem by Dylan Thomas, which contains the lines "Do not go gentle into that good night." And "Rage, rage, against the dying of the light." It's quite famous, of course. It's an homage or advice to an admired dying person, counselling him to rebel. It extolls him for not accepting or acquiescing in mortality. Instead of Buddhist or Franciscan resignation, it advocates protest. It praises him for not lying down before the unfairness of death, but demanding his civil rights, human justice.

But the older I get, and the longer I practice as a paramedic, the more dubious the poem seems. Leave aside calling that night "good." I know *goodnight* is like *goodbye*, but what else is good about it? I would have written "Do not go gently into that bad night." Of course that may be why Thomas is a great if minor poet and I'm not. No, the main problem I have with those lines is that they seem like empty bravado, just rhodomontade. He's going to die anyway. How admirable is it, really, for him to make his last days a misery for his caretakers and family? I mean, he has the right, and they should just put up with it and shut up. A medic with a difficult hospice patient is just a medic doing his job. He shouldn't whine about it. He should just exercise some understanding. But that doesn't make the rager is someone I necessarily want to emulate. He might be just a burnt out alcoholic poet with multiple serious psych issues. Anger management problems is something I'm very familiar with from own life as well as my patients'. It's narcissistic. Many times, I should have just kept my mouth shut, even when I was facing an injustice, which was not always even the case. I mean, who doesn't? Death, for example. Maybe the people I was pissed at had their own injustices to face.

I now think it's a young, romantic poet's poem. He thinks we have an indomitable spirit in a dying body. Actually, in real life, the spirit declines as quickly or even more quickly than "the body."

But my hero, Ben, the terrorist, that's another matter. He took up arms against a sea of troubles. Staff was not treating him right. And then they were ignoring his justified complaints against official oppression. Not unlikely they were laying hands on him. Changing his diaper or his clothes. Perhaps preventing him from getting up from his bed or wheelchair; surely, not allowing him to leave. In the outside world, this would be called assault and battery, kidnapping, false imprisonment, bullying, persecution. Official oppression.

Did he whine uselessly? Rage against the dying of the light? No, he seized the only opportunity to defend himself. Despite his physical weakness, advanced age, deteriorating mental faculties, he made like James Bond. Except in real life. Attacked from all sides, at bay like the panting hart beset by hounds, he adroitly extricated himself. Bruce Lee could have done no better. He used the milliseconds available to him, brilliantly devining the strategy which would enable him to defeat a more powerful, better armed and more numerous enemy, all in their youth and in full possession of mental and physical powers. Consummate professionals, where he was only an amateur, improvising against their well trained and experienced hands.

He wrestled the fire extinguisher from the wall; he set his back against the corner, where he knew he could not be flanked, despite his small and waning numbers. He turned and fired. He directed his nozzle, despite being unfamiliar with the weapon, against his horde of persecutors, like Rambo or that woman in Aliens. He sprayed their asses but good.

Like Terminator 2, he avoided all casualties, except himself, and then only a flesh wound.

Despite their best malevolent attempts, none of the masses arrayed against him could dislodge him from his purely defensive position until he had exhausted his only weapon. Our response took more than 5 minutes, and his slow witted persecutors probably didn't even call us until they saw that their own futile and malign attempts were getting nowhere, so he had his back to the wall, and his surgically precise sniping protecting him, for at least 15 minutes.

It may not seem like a long time, but neither is 93 years.

"Freedom," he shouted. "Free at last! Thank God Almighty, I'm free at last! If I have only one, brief life, let me live it as a free man!"

WELL, GAG ME WITH A SPOON

We were dispatched to a trailer park for an unresponsive patient. It was a decent kind of park, green, shaded, attractive, with well spread out homes and respectable residents, the same park where I had been threatened by John Wayne (may he rest in peace) just the week before.

That week it had been for shortness of breath. We had rolled through the trees and a nice meadow to the address, and then stepped up the front stairs into a very large living area, considering it was a trailer home. A double wide. A middle aged guy was standing there panting. He was not overly obese, considering it was San Antonio, but his color was not great. Nothing remarkable, he just didn't look healthy. As always, I was alert to the area around me when walking into a scene, and now I had the sensation someone was behind me. I turned, and sure enough, there was. With a gun. Big gun.

It was John Wayne.

Life size, too, on the biggest TV screen I had ever seen. John being, unfortunately, beyond my help, despite his healthy appearance, and not dangerous, I turned back to my patient and put a stethoscope on his chest. He was breathing at 30, a little fast, but only mildly labored, and his lungs were clear as a bell. So that meant cardiac to me, and we handled it like an acute cardiac. That is, if he was out of breath, but his lungs were working fine, and his CO_2 and pulse oximetry were OK, it indicated that it was likely the pump that was not working. Or maybe a pulmonary embolism, possibly.

This time, though, we were met at another trailer, a single wide, by a trim, muscular, good looking Hispanic man in his 40's. He stepped back from his front door to indicate a woman with long dark hair, also 40ish, lying in the middle of his living room floor. She was also trim, wearing shorts and a tank top, with good color, no visible indication of any health problems, but she was unconscious. Not a deep coma, about a Glasgow 7, but her main problem was breathing, which she was barely doing.

Rather than bother with any further assessment or vitals—these could wait--my partner had pulled out the intubation kit, and she now began handing me a MAC 3 laryngoscope—my favorite blade--and the 7 mm endotracheal tube I asked for. 7: middle sized adult female. She had already threaded the stylette into it. I checked to be sure it was the adult one and not the infant one, which doesn't give you enough stiffness to get into the trachea. I know because I once tried on a full arrest. A newbie had put in the wrong stylette. Slowed me up substantially until I figured out what was wrong.

I bent this one into the hockey stick shape I like, got my partner to put one hand under the base of the patient's neck and lift, and her other hand to press on the cricoid. This was all a little tense, of course, but I had been intubating someone in the field about once every other month, so I was getting used to it. Besides, the patient was still breathing, if not a lot. And we hadn't run into any problems yet.

Mac 4 is probably the most popular laryngoscope blade. It's small and handy but not too small. It has a neat curved shape, so you can lift the tongue up after just going into the valecula right under the base of the tongue. You don't have to stick it all the way down the throat and then back it out till the vocal cords pop into view, as you have to do with the straight, Miller blade. Which also doesn't hold the tongue out of the way as well.

I did hear a doc call the Mac 3 "a woman's blade" once. I was OK with that. I always figured I must have a feminine side to my nature somewhere.

With the patient's head now tipped back, with me squatting above her head, facing down her body, I slid the laryngoscope into her mouth below her tongue, lifted straight up, and got a magnificent view of her vocal cords. With my right hand I then slid my ET tube between them. I put it in pretty deep, well past the little black mark suitable for in-hospital intubations. You have to check that you have not gone too far, into the right main stem bronchus, but since we move intubated patients, you really like to get that tube in there secure, much farther than ER docs seem to be comfortable with. Then I held the tube in place with my left hand, and pulled my stethoscope from around my neck with the right. My partner had by then attached the bag valve mask (BVM), already hooked to oxygen, to the protruding end of the ET tube, and begun bagging. I listened for breath sounds over both lungs. Both lungs sounded like wheezy BVM—no main stem intubation. Then I listened to the stomach, just to the right of midline epigastric, which is where the stomach is. Not in the middle.

Nice and quiet. No esophageal intubation either. The ET tube misted on the exhales, oxygen SATs and CO_2 capnography continued to be excellent. I tied the tube down and inflated its cuff with the syringe my partner handed me.

One time I was trying to listen like this, and the nurse on scene, who was bagging, stopped so I could hear better. "BVM," I snapped. Her word for it was ambu-bag so she needed more nudging. Since the patient was not breathing, if the BVM was not going, there would be nothing at all to hear. Obviously. The thing is really noisy, fortunately, so it's really easy to hear it squawking through the lungs.

Back to our patient. She was a really easy tube. No gag reflex either, so I didn't have to paralyze her first, which would have upped the tension quite substantially.

So there we were. The patient was lying on her back, my partner was breathing for her with a bag valve mask hooked to oxygen, five breaths a minute as per protocol, and the fireman first responder had already discovered that the patient's vitals were pretty good. Stable for the time being.

We still needed to check blood sugar, pupils, and some other stuff, but first I stood up, and turned to my host to see if I could get some history or an idea as to what was going on, before we transported. The other fireman had already brought up the stretcher and backboard and c collar. We don't transport an intubated patient without them, under the theory that whatever will keep someone's cervical spine nice and straight, along the back of his neck, will also do the same for the trachea, at the front of his neck, so the tube will stay in place. The worst thing that can happen is losing the tube, most particularly if it ends up down the esophagus instead of the trachea. Dead patient and terminated medic will be your usual outcome.

I once listened to an orthopedic surgeon telling a horror story about flipping over a patient to get to the back of his neck, and losing the tube. "Aww," I said, "you had to move an intubated patient? That's tough." Try loading one on a stretcher and then transporting him in an ambulance going 93 mph, all while doing chest compressions.

If you can't get the intubation, or you lose it, and you realize that, and continue bagging with an oral airway in place, instead of the tube, that's all acceptable, if not desirable, but a tube in the wrong place is a career ender.

On the other hand, when, as always, the documenting clerk asks you what the measurement was at the lips, and you say, "I have no idea" (I mean, you got other stuff to do than document the ET tube markings at the patient's lips), that goes over fine. She looks taken aback for an instant, and then picks up your amused smile.

My host was remarkably calm for a person with an unconscious guest. I liked him. He was straightforward, good humored, open without being effusive, calm, fit, good-looking, had on nice shorts, sandals and a blue chambray shirt, everything you could want. Nice, clean, curvy muscular feet.

His story was that he had hired her to spend the night, she had shot up, and then this happened. We had not noticed any tracks. Given how healthy she looked we hadn't really suspected her of being a junkie.

In the old days, there was a 'coma cocktail' you gave to any unconscious unknown. It was thiamine, dextrose and Narcan. Thiamine is rarely used for alcoholics in the field any more, and we take blood sugars now to find out if someone really needs dextrose before we administer it. We take the blood sugar for any altered mental state, for stroke symptoms, in fact on every medical patient and many traumas (WHY did they wreck their car?), much less coma. So, unfortunately, the Narcan sometimes gets forgotten too. Narcan reverses opiates. It's an opiate antagonist.

I was once on a call with a reasonably good medic, when I was still in training, who barely managed to get a patient to the ER alive, because she had had such a struggle to keep her breathing with the bag valve mask the entire transport. She had not intubated, as the patient had a gag, and she had not wanted to paralyze and intubate, I don't know why, and she had forgotten the Narcan. The patient was a 55 year old middle class respectable housewife, found in nice suburban home with absolutely no indication she was on opiate medications or took heroin, but it turned out she had fibromyalgia or some other chronic pain condition, and someone had prescribed Methadone for it. She took too much. She was pale, turning blue when we found her. Lots of people take opiates, is what I learned from that. Check pupils. Narcan for all.

The Doc in the ER had immediately shot Narcan into her, so she was sitting up, breathing well, good color and fully conscious, no acute distress, within a minute. The medic was pissed with me for not driving well, too rough and not fast enough. This was true enough, it being one of my first emergency transports as driver, but, looking back on it, that was hardly the main problem.

I've also learned over the years not to reverse opiate overdoses at all if the patient is breathing OK and has stable vitals. If he's stable, let him stay sedated. He's nice and safe. And not bouncing off the ambulance walls, or attempting to throttle me because I've returned him, bright eyed, bushy tailed, fanged and fisted, to a world he does not approve of, and was successfully avoiding, until I interfered.

Hardly chagrined about having missed tracks—we had just started our exam—we shoved some Narcan down the IV, which was my next intervention. Just 1 mg to start with. Junkies are hard to get IVs into, usually. You can get the needle in all right, but then it won't thread, because the lumens of the veins are all scarred and narrowed. She had healthy veins though. Not a stone junkie.

Pretty soon—I hadn't even finished getting a history from my host, and he hardly knew anything—she opened up her eyes. She looked around with just her eyes (her head being bagged and fixed by the tube), kind of alarmed. The place was not in the same shape as when she had left it. Before, there had not been any firemen, much less medics and firemen. Backboards, c collars, jump bags and drug boxes had not been part of the décor. Her arm had not had a running IV in it. She clearly remembered removing her needle.

Most of all, there had not been a 7 mm ET tube stuck down into her airway. My partner had stopped bagging, as the patient began to breathe on her own, and thus to fight the bag valve mask. So at least no one was forcing air down her throat any more, which she vaguely remembered as part of coming out of the coma.

My partner, noticing her wide-eyed alarm and shifting eyes, asked if she would like the tube removed. She nodded. Can't speak with an ET tube between your vocal cords. My partner looked at me, I nodded too, and she deflated the cuff and pulled the tube.

And so here is kind of the most remarkable part of this story, if not the point. It was unusual but not unknown to have a patient with such a high Glasgow score and yet no gag. Most people have to be pretty close to death to lose that reflex. Glasgow 3 or maybe 4. But the fact that she could tolerate an ET tube down her trachea, even while she was fully alert and looking around the room, had to be what you might call a professional achievement or gift, like Lance Armstrong's unusually high maximum pulse rate or Arnold Schwarzenegger's muscles.

Pretty soon our patient was on her feet and declining transport. I pointed out that the Narcan doesn't last as long as the heroin, so there was a possibility she would pass out again, but she was undismayed. I'm encouraged to transport everyone, because of the liability of leaving someone on scene, but there have to be exceptions, especially when you consider that 85% of people who call 911 do not need emergent transport to a hospital, and well over half don't need an ambulance at all. Once you fix a diabetic's blood sugar, and she has a chance to eat, and a good explanation for why she crashed to start with, like she took her insulin and didn't eat anything, or threw up all her food, then you can't really find a good reason to convince her to transport. An already diagnosed epileptic who has a seizure is not going to have another one for months, likely enough, so there isn't much an emergency room MD can do for him really, except check his anti-convulsant med levels. Or the patient could just take them.

This lady did not want to go either. Given she was walking around, hale and hearty, alert and oriented, not even opiated anymore, there was nothing I could do to dissuade her from signing a refusal, with the appropriate warnings and documentation in place. Given I was going to take a signed refusal, I kind of regretted not having had her sign it while the ET tube was still in place. That would have made a heck of a picture, if I were in the habit of taking or allowed to take pictures of patients. Intubated patient signing a refusal.

Instead, after we got our 2nd set of vitals, completed our full exam (still no tracks), taken a copious history and wrote up a patient report all signed and sealed, we packed up our stuff, got back in the truck and waved goodbye. Our host and patient were strolling around their lawn next to the roadway, watching us go. They made a cute couple.

THE SOUL

As a Paramedic, my partners were mostly Basics, basic EMT. There's a definite, discernible hierarchy, not just socially, but in intelligence, width of knowledge, even subtlety of manner, as you go up the scale from Basic to Paramedic, to RN to MD; but at the same time you find the usual infinite variety of human beings. We defer to the MD—our title says we are in the service of the physician—and almost all of them deserve it. They know more, their medical reasoning is more acute; better insight and sophistication are visible even in their faces and surely language.

Many novelists like to take the position that everyone is equally subtle within, and that characters of lower education or intelligence are merely less articulate about their--actually equally nuanced--feelings and relationships. It's not true. Surely there are brilliant and subtle people who are not particularly verbal, but, generally, expression, thought and feeling go together. A person incapable of giving any kind of accurate and nuanced account of his argument with his wife usually just doesn't have an accurate and nuanced position. Or emotional experience.

Still, though, people become Basics from many directions. I was teasing an Indian Basic I met at SAMMC, saying I had never met an Indian who wasn't a physician. "Well, I'm only 18," she said plaintively. She was, in other words, on the way to becoming an MD, and working as a Basic on that route.

During the great recession, any number of college graduates filtered into the EMS business, unable and sometimes unwilling to work elsewhere. Health care was still booming.

Then, there are some really really smart people who have learning disabilities, and are unable to get ahead by the academic route. There are people of great emotional and intuitive subtlety who are not intellectual. Conversely, people who are lazy, or criminal, or feckless, or disorganized, or sick, or disturbed, or have personality disorders in their high school and early college years, may bloom late. Many Basics are, of course, on their way to Paramedic, or RN, or PA.

So I had many partners, of all kinds. I may talk about some of the really awful ones later. There were only a few, really. EMTs are nice people, in my experience. They like to help people, not only patients but the people they work with; they're conscientious, scrupulous about care, and easy to get along with, certainly compared to the academics I encountered in a previous life.

I mean, think about academics. Nerds are known for social awkwardness and self-involvement. If they manage to get a tenured position, they're *ambitious* nerds, and probably political too. Then they get arrogant about their success. To them, everyone else is a school dropout. Arrogant, ambitious, political nerds. Maybe the occasional lover of wisdom.

Instead, today I'm going to talk about an interesting partner who ended up being really illustrative about what the profession of medicine entails in terms of understanding disease processes and their effect on people's behavior and thinking.

India was a drop out from a PHD program in anthropology. She was extremely well read. She was pretty in a frail, pale way, and both physically and socially awkward, but not to a marked extent. Very liberal Austin background. Totem animal a sloth or an aye aye.

She could be quite witty. Once I choked on some of the carrot I was eating. This was the second time this happened on the same shift. After coughing vigorously, I said, "I wonder if my epiglottis works right. My Mom was always gagging on stuff too. Of course, she lived to 92 and died of breast cancer."

India said, "I'm fully confident of your ability to survive vegetables."

She wrote horror fiction, which she had some success at publishing, but wouldn't show anyone. Someone who publishes well in genre fiction, by the way, can be wildly successful financially. She was not. It may be she felt shy about showing her work, or she was embarrassed because it was nasty, repugnant and disgusting: everything horror fiction ought to be.

In fact, she viewed working as an EMT as like working in a sales or janitorial job, as an easy gig which paid enough to allow her to pursue her real interests.

Whereas I had been really nervous about making mistakes when I was a Basic, she said she wasn't. She said she figured I could handle any emergency so she didn't have to stress about the possibilities. Maybe she had a point about handling stuff on scene, but what about driving me to the right hospital in an emergency? For she was definitely directionally challenged.

What medics refer to as "Can't find her own ass with a flashlight." Or "she needs GPS to get home after work."

We were following another truck once, to give a lift assist, and we got stopped at a light. I was driving; she was navigating from the map book. Nowadays most people use the GPS on their phone, which means, unfortunately, that they have no fucking idea where they are. India told me to turn right instead of left onto the correct street. Apparently she had thought we were going North when we were going South. "I wondered why the streets were coming up in backwards order," she said.

This was one of the reasons I went straight through to Paramedic instead of working as a Basic for a while, which might have been better. Driving my paramedic to the hospital made me more nervous than handling the patient in the back

This was the beginning of my problems with her. That is, we got along fine on the job, but without real rapport. Because I take my job really seriously. I work hard at it and I believe I have a gift for it. I take pride in my work. I understand writers taking jobs as cabbies or janitors, but if they want to take advantage of the long posting periods and down times at quiet EMS stations, I still expect them to bend every sinew to save lives when a call does come.

India was conscientious enough but she treated patients like customers. Now, we're in a service profession, and transport agencies don't get called by the facility if staff doesn't like the way the medic acts, so this served pretty well most of the time, but being an EMT is still different from being a salesperson in a clothing store.

She would for example ask a demented patient, "Would it be OK if I take your blood pressure?"

Now, this sounds very thoughtful, but what do you do if he says "No!" People with dementia don't merely have cognitive problems. The sweet old lady who is totally disoriented is rare indeed. Most people with dementia also have serious emotional and character breakdowns. Just being disoriented puts a person in a fearful and bad mood by itself, even if the emotive parts of his brain aren't breaking down as well.

The issue here is that a person who is alert and oriented X 4, to person, place, time and event, who can answer the four questions (what is your name/ where are you/ what year is it/ what happened) can refuse care. If he's bleeding to death or having a heart attack or driving his wheelchair in traffic, he has a right to do that, as long as he doesn't admit to being suicidal by word or act.

But someone who is non compos mentis cannot consent to or decline medical care. His care becomes your responsibility. You have to take care of him the way you believe he would want if he were rational, the way you would want to be taken care of, assuming you're rational.

So there India was. This guy was sick. Had to get a BP. But she's staring at him, paralyzed.

In those situations I say, "I'm going to take your blood pressure. It doesn't hurt. Hold still." You want to be nice and keep him in the loop as much as possible, but you need a BP, hook or crook. Put a cuff on by force if necessary and then distract him or hold him down till it reads. If he's not really sick, you can let it go, but it's like kids. If they're not in extremis, I won't put in an IV if they don't really need it. Let them suffer the pain of a broken humerus instead of getting IV pain killer, if they refuse, terrified of needles. And they are.

The very last thing I would ever put up with is hurting a kid. But if he needs an IV, or a diabetic with altered mental status needs IV glucose, or a demented person needs suction, I take real pleasure (Freud might say sadistic pleasure) in rescuing them by force, getting that IV in their wriggling arm while a fireman is holding them down. It's a sport with real life consequences and rewards.

And indeed, even worse, India'd ask a guy who was aspirating vomit or fluids if it was OK to suction. Now, no one likes being suctioned. Makes you gag. But you must do it, by force if necessary. It's either gagging on your Yankauer suction cath, or aspiration pneumonia, which old people often do not survive. Or no airway at all, which is fatal in three minutes.

I took the Yank out of her hand, grabbed the old guy by the head, and ran it around his mouth until I effected entry, namely via a missing tooth, where I could slide it in despite his clenched teeth. Make no mistake about it, this was brutal, and yet it was probably "another life saved."

India said "that was brilliant" about the missing tooth maneuver, but she didn't have that quite right either. I do not think to myself, "Hey, this guy is old, he probably has a missing tooth somewhere, so I can use the space to get the Yank down his throat," any more than a point guard knows there's going to be a path to the basket, or a boxer sees a gap before he puts his fist through it. I think with my hands. There's nothing very special about this. All point guards drive, all boxers punch, and all medics will do whatever they can to clear a compromised airway. Some are better at it than others, obviously.

When I walk into her room, I often know what a patient has and how serious it is even before I do the exam. India just did not have this clinical instinct. I don't know if it was some residual nominalism or residue of Christianity--she was not religious—but she could not get it out of her head that somewhere down there under a patient's incoherence, confusion, semi-consciousness, disease, dementia, there was still a fully conscious alert human being, just like herself. Underneath the dementia, inside the coma, was a fully intact soul, somewhere.

Now, everyone starts as a newbie. One of the big surprises when you get out of class onto the street is that they really expect you to do all this stuff. Intubate, shock, paralyze, revive dead people, deliver babies. ("Don't worry, ma'am. I read the chapter twice.") But I wasn't sure India was even trying.

Probably the best example would be the lady we took to her doctor's appointment from her nursing home. Betsy was about 45, disheveled, unkempt, talkative, emotional, obese, and she had end stage liver disease, cirrhosis. We were taking her to her liver transplant specialist for some medical problems she had developed.

The MD was alert, personable, friendly, obviously very smart, and willing to talk to us about this patient. Wool skirt, open warm face, brown eyes. She told Betsy flat out that she was not a candidate for transplant, and that she would not be seeing her anymore. She was transferring care to the nursing home MD.

Betsy began wailing. She demanded to be taken to another hospital where she could see another doctor.

India was distraught too.

Betsy had no history of alcohol abuse, so I asked the Doc what had caused the cirrhosis. "Obesity," she said. Plain and simple. The story was that Betsy had destroyed her liver simply by being too fat. Fatty liver. She wasn't huge by our standards but she did weigh well over 200 lbs at 5'5". Over the last few years her doctors had hooked her up with nutritionists, therapists, and told her repeatedly that her obesity was morbid. Betsy had not succeeded in losing weight. It was questionable whether she had even tried. Now she had hepatic encephalopathy, meaning that the poisons her liver was failing to filter out of her blood were damaging her brain. She was equivalent to demented. Labile, emotional, poor short term memory, lapses in memory, mood, temper. Not unlikely, she had been bipolar or something even before, and perhaps this was why she had been noncompliant.

You like some patients and don't like others. You behave professionally in any case, but it's just a fact of life. This has been shown to affect pain management, and you wonder how much else. And it's individual and influenced by circumstances. How late in the shift it is, whether your partner is feckless and has been getting on your nerves.

I did not like Betsy at all. Her willful helplessness, ditzy emotionality, the sloppy obesity, just struck me the wrong way. In general, patients who just cart themselves to the MD, as if to the beauty parlor, and make it his responsibility to care for them, or even to know about their conditions, irritate me. I try hard myself to be responsible and knowledgeable about my health, and other people's. It's not easy, and sometimes it seems like it's one of the few things I can do well. So I'm not always tolerant of people who don't even try.

Generally I feel compassion and sympathy for my patients; some of them really appeal to me, but there are exceptions. I hope I'm professional enough so they don't realize it. And the ones I don't like are generally so narcissistic that they probably don't notice much about how I feel anyway. Though there are people who combine idiocy, irresponsibility, incompetence and utter disregard for other people, with acute sensitivity to how they're being treated.

So at this point the MD was not going to give her a new liver. There are only so many to go around. Transplant specialists ration them to patients who will gain the most benefit. Betsy already had deteriorating mentation, which was incurable even with a new liver. She had been noncompliant even before she had lost impulse control, perseverance and planning ability, along with her liver and brain.

Betsy continued to wail, understandably. She understood, at least for the moment, that she was being condemned to die a slow and miserable death over the next months. Liver failure. Even a good death is ugly and unjust, and this was not going to be a good death.

India however did not get it. She was not only sympathetic, but determined to help. On our way back to Betsy's nursing home bed, India stopped the stretcher by the front office and demanded to see the social worker. Politely, as always.

The social worker came out of her office, kind of nonplussed, and obviously pretty busy. There's never anywhere near enough staff in these facilities, what with cutbacks, and the low level of support for mental health and social services to start with.

The front offices and entryway were immaculate, decorated in a professional, McMansion kind of way, as they always are, even when the rest of the facility is low rent, which this one was not. Squeaky clean, shiny polished tile floors, artificial plants, tastefully low key art work on the walls, well-dressed professional staff persons.

We introduced Betsy to her social worker, who pretty clearly already had to know Betsy.

"This is Sally, your social worker," we said. "Any questions you have about your care or about your doctors you can ask to see her, and ask her. Remember that name. Sally."

The social worker took this in good spirit, though she was, as I said, nonplussed.

We took Betsy to her bedroom. All kinds of personal knick knacks and photos, kind of disorderly actually. Moved her to her bed via draw sheet, tucked her in.

"So, Betsy," I said. "Who is your social worker?"

"What?"

"What is the name of your social worker?"

"What, why are you asking me? Are you asking me a question?"

"No, I'm making a point."

Betsy looked confused.

"I get it," India said.

I don't believe she did.

MY BOSS

I've mentioned my boss, Sally Dick, several times. Besides being a character, she's a notable figure in EMS, surely worthy of a chapter or more. Sally is the founder and CEO of Retro Ambulance, which she started 20 years ago with just a couple trucks, and has built up to be the major provider of ambulance services for city of over 2 million people, not to mention surrounding areas.

Legend has it, she used to field ambulance requests on her unit cell phone, in the back of her ambulance, while taking care of a patient at the same time. Before she was a paramedic, she was a cop.

She worked 911 in the wild and wooly days before there was as much supervision or equipment. Once she had to crawl across a dentist's lawn to drag him to safety, while the cops distracted his wife, still in the house and still armed. He had been having an affair and she put a stop to it with a 9 milllimeter. He didn't survive. She had managed to put more than half the magazine into him.

Sally is a 6 ft redhead with green eyes and a killer figure. On the 4 inch stilettos she liked to wear around the office, she should have been eye level with me, though it always seemed I was standing in a pit, somehow. Like confronting a lighthouse except it moved and yelled. She is loud, colorful, generous, funny, witty, has a genius intelligence level, and a hair trigger. An incisive writer and speaker, one of her main gifts is her ability to penetrate to the gist or heart of a situation virtually instantaneously, and articulate a solution in the next heartbeat.

Her take on the problems I've described having with facility staff is "Semon is a good medic, but he's not suave." Suave. An uncommon word, but really apt. Sums up pages of my narration with a single, well-chosen word.

Everyone in the Texas EMS community knows her. Given her strong personality, not all of them like her, by any means, but more do, and all of them respect her.

I'm not going to discuss her business model, which I don't fully understand anyway, but I will tell a couple of stories which I know about from my own observation.

We transported a patient from a rehab center to SAMMC orthopedic clinic for a follow up checkup. This woman was slight, dark haired and fucked up. In several senses. She had caused a motor vehicle accident by some ditzy maneuver of her own doing, and its principal victim had been herself. Probably not wearing a seatbelt, she had gone "down and under" and trashed her legs.

SAMMC surgeons, trauma and orthopedic, had put her back together again by means of external fixators, among other devices. This meant that for her rehab period she lay in bed with her legs bolted back together with braces and pins exterior to the skin, and penetrating through it to her bones, which they were holding in place so they could heal properly. SAMMC was treating her pro bono, as a service to the public, because she had no insurance or support system, certainly not one capable of dealing with multiple surgeries and follow up rehab.

Among other complications, mental and physical, she was HIV positive.

We found the Ortho clinic in SAMMC's maze without too much difficulty, having been there before.

We presented ourselves to the sergeant who was the charge nurse. He sent us to the back of the line, stating that just because she came in an ambulance didn't mean our patient got priority over anyone else.

Well, fair enough in one sense, but, as Sally put it, Retro Ambulance provides transport, not in-hospital care. I gave her a call for instructions. Days when calls are light, she will let a truck and crew sit with a patient in a facility for some time. Days when other patients need her trucks, she will give the facility only 20 minutes, tops, to accept the patient. If not, they go back to their nursing home, or wherever they came from, and someone reschedules.

This was one of the busy days, or one when Sally was not feeling excessively patient. She told us 20 more minutes, then leave.

The patient started to cry. "My ankle really hurts, it has for two days, and I know something is wrong. I have to see the doctor!"

"OK, I'll let you talk to the charge nurse yourself, but we can't stay here any longer. My boss needs us to go take care of some other people."

I braved the head of the line again with the stretcher, and my patient got her moment of fame with the charge nurse. His position was that they had no beds available for her.

I didn't say anything, but my thought was, SAMMC is a 500 bed hospital. I have one stretcher. They need my stretcher?

"Well," he said to us, relenting, "she's alert and oriented? Stable?"

"Absolutely," I said.

"OK, if she doesn't need any supervision, I guess we can find a gurney for her to wait on."

We transferred her to his gurney, handed over her voluminous documentation and our paperwork, cleared, and went on to the next call.

I did hear the rest of the story this time, and it went like this.

Everything was going fine, she was waiting patiently, when she developed a nose bleed. Staff was tied up putting pressure and bandages on her nose. They were already unhappy about this situation even before they found out she was HIV positive.

Sally got a call from the sergeant. "Your crew never told us she was HIV positive!" he exclaimed, concluding his tirade about the situation. Now, this was true enough in one sense. He had not taken or wanted any kind of full report, just a few words. Too busy, he had just accepted her paperwork. Which absolutely did report her HIV status.

"Sir, do you mean to tell me," Sally said, "that you failed to take universal precautions for BLOOD? Is that what you're trying to tell me?"

One of Sally's business secrets is that what she looks for in a medic, basic or paramedic, is attitude. Appearance counts. She wants her staff to look professional in their grooming and dress. No beards for example. But above all, attitude. She feels she can work on the other aspects of their practice, but that one is the base. Sometimes when you're trying to explain something to her, you sense she's just listening with half an ear. Most of her attention is focused on whether your uniform, matching undershirt and boots are up to snuff.

A good illustration would be the week she fired two crew members and rescued another.

What happened was that one crew was posted in an outlying town to provide coverage for her contract facilities there. The crew had called out which restaurant they were going to be in, as per protocol. She does not want crews hanging out in her truck when they are not using it. She does not want them running the engine to stay cool in the air-conditioning. So Earn Money Sleeping is not the Retro way of EMS. She's said, reasonably, "I don't mind someone dozing off, but no lying down horizontal on the job. Doesn't look professional. "

Well, these two gentleman not only were sleeping in the truck, and in the front seat, perfectly visible to all and sundry, but they were actually to be found across the street from where they had said they were going to be.

When they awoke, someone from the restaurant told them that someone in uniform had come and taken their picture while they were asleep. Reading the handwriting on the wall, they brought their pagers, ID and extra uniforms with them when they came in the next day.

The person who had photographed them was the on duty supervisor. She told me she was fully prepared to accept an apology and a reasonable explanation with suitable remorse, but instead, the medic said, "Well, we were posted there for 4 hours. Of course we're going to sleep. I worked 70 hours already this week and had a structure fire last night at my fire job to boot."

So indeed they received walking papers.

But the interesting part is what also happened that same week. Sally was driving by a McDonald's where one of her trucks was posted. She looked inside and saw one of her medics there. So she parked and walked over to her truck. And started banging on the side.

The other medic crawled out, rubbing his eyes.

"What are you doing sleeping in my truck? Why aren't you inside with your partner?"

"I'm really sorry, but I don't have any money," the medic said sheepishly. "I won't do it again. I swear."

So Sally gave him 20 bucks and sent him inside.

It's all about attitude.

Among the many reasons I would not be able to run an
ambulance company (more are discussed below) is that I'm kind
of slow when it comes to business relationships. Clueless might
be the word. I'm not suave, in Sally's formulation. The long
game is not my forte. I win battles and lose wars. I'm a
paramedic.

It doesn't help that I can't remember people's names or faces
either. So I needed quite a bit of nudging when it came to the
problem with St Peter's Hospital, Central Hospital and the psych
facility where this particular patient originated.

We had been called code three, emergent, for a patient
presenting with, supposedly, bradycardia, hypotension and
altered mental status. However, when I evaluated the patient, I
found her to be only mildly bradycardic, which was easily
explained by the BP med she was taking; not really hypotensive
at all, and, as for altered mental, well, she was a psych patient.
She was lethargic, stating she had not been able to sleep for
three days, but when you aroused her she could answer the
four questions perfectly fine.

So I was transporting her to the distant hospital the psych
facility had requested, St Peter's, non-emergent. She just
looked pretty good to me, her color, muscle tone, breathing not
indicating a problem that was going to be an imminent threat to
life or limb.

But when I called it in to St Peter's, the receiving RN stated
that she thought this patient ought to go emergent to the
nearest appropriate facility. Now, she had a perfect right to
bump me up to priority one. She also had a perfect right to
divert me to another facility.

But what slipped my mind—this is what we call a brain fart in EMS—is that she did not have a right to send me to *another* hospital lights and sirens. That is, as soon as she diverted me from her hospital, the patient became my sole charge again, in my ambulance, under my care. It was up to me to decide whether I should bring her in emergent or non-emergent.

However, apparently this was too subtle for me at the time. So I diverted to Central Hospital. Priority One. Lights and sirens. Now, of course if the patient had turned out to be circling the drain, and I had elected to transport her non-emergent, that would have been quite a problem for me. Not to say the patient. Especially if it came out an RN had advised me to run hot.

But that wasn't the case. My problem turned out to be the opposite, the receiving nurse at Central asking me why I had brought in this stable patient priority one. It did not help that I agreed with her. Nor that my only explanation was that a nurse at St Peter's, who had never seen the patient, and had nothing to do with the patient, had thought she was critical.

"Well, see, yeah, I agree she's stable, but this nurse over at St Peter's—no, I didn't get her name--no, the patient came from the psych facility, not St Peter's--see, she thought that, well—so how did she know? Yes, that's a good question!"

Sally wasn't pleased either but for another reason. The psych facility had requested St Peter's, and yet I had brought the patient to Central, and didn't have any kind of good reason for doing so, as the patient was surely stable enough to be transported to the more distant facility requested.

I had a good excuse for that one though. The nurse at St Peter's had diverted me. I could over-ride her diversion, but only in the case where I was bringing in someone emergent who

I believed had to go to that hospital. So in this case I had no excuse or reason to over-ride her diversion.

So Sally called St Peter's. She had quite an argument with them. She said, "You keep trying to get me to transport patients to your facility, and then when I do, you refuse her.

"I know your RN decided she was too critical to come that far, but the medic bringing her in has 11 years of experience, he's a good medic and he didn't think so, and neither did Central, when we finally had to bring her there."

Well, it turns out the RN had 17 years of experience, and was an RN, not a paramedic....

The upshot of this was that I was kind of persona non grata at St Peters for months after that. Now, there were other issues too, to be sure. I had failed to hand over a face sheet to the clerk fast enough for his taste when I brought in an emergent patient, and I hadn't been overly friendly about his officiousness, either, being focused on the critical patient rather than the paperwork. That was easy enough to straighten out. I found out that none of the orders for lab work etc. for the patient can be filled until she is registered, so the clerk was just doing his job, kind of over and above actually. He still shouldn't have been rude, but I should have made allowances for his assiduousness.

Afterwards I had to explain to Sally why I had diverted etc.

"But Sally," I said, "you told me to be polite and deferential to the staff at facilities, and to just do what they want, no argument." See, I had been chewed out in the past for arguing with staff about what I thought was best for their patient.

The background here is that we have a saying in paramedicine, "treat the patient, not the monitor." That is, if the monitor shows the patient to have a shockable rhythm or severe bradycardia or the like, but the patient looks perfectly fine, we should go by the patient condition, not what the monitor is saying. Either it's incorrect or account has to be taken of how well this particular patient is tolerating a condition which might be lethal for someone else.

Well, at Retro, the saying has been adapted to, "treat the facility, not the patient." As Sally once patiently explained, the patients do not call us, the facilities do. If the facility doesn't like us, we get no calls, even if our patient care was excellent.

Now this is not a matter of giving poor patient care. We still do our best. It's a matter of tact, of keeping your mouth shut, of working within what the circumstances allow. Do what you need to do in your truck.

It can be tricky, though, particularly if the patient needs something on scene which we don't even carry in the truck, like insulin. 911 work was more straightforward. It's just you and the patient. Everyone else has to get out of the way. They are not going to call another 911 next time, and how many next times will there be anyway? They can complain, but a well-connected director will investigate, and support you if you were right.

So in this case I just thought I was learning my lesson and being appropriately deferential to facility staff when I accepted the RN's recommendation.

"Semon," Sally said, barely suppressing 'you dummy.' "St Peter's is not one of our contracts. You can be as mean as you like to them!"

And the psych facility in question was one of our contracts, you see. It's too bad for me that paramedicine isn't just about taking care of one patient at a time. I would prefer a world which was somewhat less complicated. Or rather where all the complications are in one field of focus, and unpleasant surprises are not blindsiding you from unexpected directions. I don't have Sally's speed of foot.

ENTREPENEUR

Well, it wouldn't be fair not to note some negatives. I'll give Sally the benefit of the doubt and frame the issues from her side by calling them aspects of the entrepreneurial spirit. That is, I live in a state, Texas, or you might say a state of mind, conservative middle America, where entrepreneurs are much admired. They are supposed to innovate, to create jobs.

So Sally is an entrepreneur all right. She started a small business and grew it into a middle sized one, and sold the whole shebang for a reputed 7 figures. You hear 12 million, you hear 25 million. She isn't saying. Some in the know say "nowhere near that," but it is in the millions.

Now, someone like Steve Jobs is innovating and creating jobs. Was Sally innovating? She had some good ideas which improved practices, like having porters making 10$ an hour wash and stock the trucks as their sole responsibility, rather than tired medics coming off their 24 hr shifts, working, slowly, erratically, on overtime. Other than that she figured out how to cut corners to save money. The equipment was all in working order and kept that way, but it was usually the cheapest available. The same can be said for the training and protocols, unfortunately. Nothing over the top fancy or up to date.

That was about it for innovation. It was a tight ship, but not a new ship.

As for creating jobs, all of these medics would have been transporting patients for another company if not hers. Sally did not create the patients or Medicare.

Would they have had worse or better jobs? Her place was clean, orderly and well organized. She did offer flexible schedules to some people and health care insurance to ones with 6 years seniority. I was able to work reduced hours, still at full time, when I got to retirement age. 36 hrs a week is practically unemployed by EMS standards. When she sold her company she made a point of insisting her staff would retain their salaries and seniority at the new place.

But her medics were for the most part financially worse off than they would have been working for Acadian or AMR, the big companies. Those companies' pay rate was the same, but they did not take medics off the clock for an hour at a time when they were posted: which cost medics thousands of bucks a year due to lost overtime. The fringes and health care and training were all better and cheaper at the bigger companies.

And then there was her temper, which seemed to get worse over time. Someone who is a perfectionist can be forgiven for expecting people to adhere to the standards she sets for herself, but then why the less than ideal training and equipment on her part?

I didn't much mind getting yelled at or sworn at, but this is the Bible Belt. Some people were quite offended. That is, it made me feel bad, but often I felt I deserved it, and the fact that it was intemperate and public, well, that was just her way. I like people to be outspoken.

Still, over time, it was the relentless negativity which got to me. Very hard to get praise and far too easy to get a rocket. I remember stepping out of the truck when I came in one night with a discarded ginseng tea can in my hand. Open containers were not allowed in the truck, but I had poured the contents into my travel mug, and was just throwing away the spent can. Sally hit the roof. My partner had to explain that I had not been drinking out of the can, but the sealed travel mug. I was hemming and hawing myself, because I was kind of thrown by the vehemence. I figured she must be talking about something more serious which I had missed.

This is kind of trivial. I mention it because it was typical. All kinds of things got Sally mad and not much made her happy, especially those final months when Retro was winding down. I can attribute it to exhaustion and burn out maybe. 24/7/365 in charge of Retro Ambulance.

Things came to a head for me personally when I finally refused a call, after making it clear for years that I did not want to work more than 12 hours a shift, barring an emergency or some other unusual circumstance. This one was a simple med eval for a psych patient, non emergent, in fact upgraded from a wheelchair van call, but her dispatcher tarted it up to pretend it was emergent, after promising me I'd get off on time, "barring an emergency." She was under a lot of pressure from Sally too.

Sally went nuclear. I mean if an errant soft drink can could get her going, imagine refusing a call. She was threatening to compromise my transition to the new company she had sold to, was saying she should complain to Texas Dept of Health, and get them to pull my patch. She was grabbing at any pot or pan to chuck at me, accusing me of lack of compassion, which had never been and was not an issue here, and of laziness.

A 67 year old guy working 12 hour shifts when he could be retired is lazy? Who worked 58 hours a week most of his career? While riding a racing bike 150 miles a week and publishing books?

Or, speaking of compassion, is firing and threatening a guy who has worked hard for you for seven years, and who you just praised to the skies to his forthcoming new boss, is that an example of compassion?

I had to sit still and listen to a full hour's worth of this. Can't argue with your boss, if she's threatening to queer the deal with your new employer.

For me it's unseemly being a boss. Everyone will laugh at your jokes, defer to your opinions. Partly it's insincere, and partly it's people's natural admiration for successful people, or an honest reaction to someone with enough charisma, after all, to have gotten to that position. But how do you know which is which? And it surely does give someone ample and probably irresistible opportunity to bully. No checks and balances in this governance.

Sally's business model, of requiring a lot of overtime from her full timers, rather than hiring more people, was kind of par for the course for EMS, and perhaps US business in general, but everyone was getting tired, and medics' morale and spirits were in decline.

Sally told me once she thought French people were lazy, after I came back from a vacation there. They did not work 48, 60, even 70 hours a week like her staff. They got holidays off and 5 weeks of vacation, rather than none and none, like her employees. She praised the loyalty and hard work of her people, just about with tears in her eyes.

Well, yes. They were making her a lot of money. Were they able to get some exercise, eat right, spend time with their families, get on with their educations? Some of them, the ones with unusual drive and energy.

To be fair, being a basic or a paramedic is not a bad job by US standards for someone with a high school education. Basics with a couple months' training were making 12$ an hour, while minimum wage was barely over 8, and McDonald's was paying 10. And EMS was more rewarding and interesting work. Paramedics were making from 16 to over 20, depending on seniority and experience. Nowadays it takes three years and $6K to get your red patch, but when I started it was a year and 1200.

They can make very decent money, but only by putting in a lot of overtime.

All the same, it would have been nice of Sally to reward her loyal and hard working employees at least with their accrued vacation pay, or better yet a little bonus of some kind, when she walked off with her millions. She did make sure they all received the same salary and seniority with the new company.

But then, having been to Europe, I'm aware of a tradition in which entrepreneurs are thought of as people who relentlessly care about one thing: making a lot of money for themselves. And for not being overly particular about who they have to squeeze or exploit to get it.

Realistically I would put Sally somewhere in between, in the real world, not some theory. She certainly did care about her employees, but abusive parents often love their kids. Power is an ugly thing. I can say myself that I have not always been as good a parent as I should have been. I yelled at my son too much. He could be a pain in the butt, but yelling didn't help. So it turns out I couldn't even run a small family without excess yelling. But that still doesn't make yelling a good thing or even an effective strategy.

Sally worked with people's schedules, she offered long timers healthcare, she kept the shop orderly, clean and well organized and she has a huge amount of charisma and business sense. On the down side, we got yelled at to the point where that was what we expected; we got penny pinched, nickeled and dimed, and bullied. I netted somewhere in the 20s for 48 weeks of 36 hours a week that last bad year. If you do the math it should have been 31k. Sure it was just post retirement age gravy, but still. Medics' protocols were not kept up to date or entrained. But perhaps that's what it takes to get a bunch of high school graduates to pull together enough to make you a successful entrepreneur. She was responsible for patients' lives, her family business, employees' jobs and, it turns out, her own health. It makes her energy even more impressive and the struggle even harder to imagine. So the uphill struggle we all witnessed was even steeper than we imagined. I could not have started or run Retro, nor would I want to. But someone has to start new businesses. In short, I'm in over my head, and also skirting a book I don't want to write. Quite an epic could be made out of Sally's uphill climb constructing a successful business, including material on economic conditions, how her relations with her employees and even family were affected, a kind of modern Buddenbrooks. Or on the other hand a better treatise could be composed about the economics of EMS and its relationship to the medical insurance quagmire. Older hands who have switched companies often respond to questions about their new employer by saying "Ah, they're all the same. One is better in some ways, the other in other ways. It just depends on what your peeves are."

Most of us have enjoyed the transition to the new company, where we get better pay, better equipment, better fringe benefits, better training and and less yelling. But also more mess and disorganization, it has to be said. And a lot more buck passing and procrastination. Plus the electronics are a disaster. CAD: computer assisted despair.

So, in a spirit of compromise, Sally, I congratulate the French on their cuisine, architecture, beautiful country, roads, cities, towns and villages, arts, culture and livable life style, on their family values, including the support given working mothers; and you on your success. Now I want to be even handed and not get into politics or economics, so it has to be said that the unemployment rate in France is 10% rather than 5% like here.

Still, are you better off unemployed there, or in that lowest five per cent here? Maybe morally: a man has to work.

So, I hope you enjoy your millions in good health, Sally. And I personally would gratefully accept a Fuji SL racing bike for my going away present, after 7 years of hard work. Sally?

GOT YOUR BACK

One of our most cherished street creds is "got your back." Another saying is, "Paramedics save lives; Basics save paramedics." That is, a strong Basic will keep his head up and try to avert mistakes before they happen.

I've always said that, in some ways, the Basic runs the full arrest. Though you can't say that to a Basic who has no subtlety of reasoning. That is, the paramedic is extremely busy. He's getting IV access, putting in a series of drugs at 3 to 5 minute intervals, calculating dosages, intubating, putting on pacing pads, checking the monitor for the heart rhythm, the capnography for CO_2 changes, trying to remember the correct algorithm fully and completely, trying not to forget to check blood sugar or to put in Narcan, deciding on bicarbonate, maybe checking pupils if he has time. Sometimes it's only the Basic who has time to see whether the fireman is doing chest compressions well enough or needs relief or counselling. Sometimes only the Basic can catch something the medic has missed or is doing wrong. Though of course the Basic is pretty busy himself, spiking an IV bag, handing up drugs and intubation equipment, putting the stylette in the ET tube, telling firemen what equipment needs to be brought from the truck, like c collars and backboards for intubated patients who are being transported.

Cliff, my first partner on a 911 post, saved my ass numerous times. In fact he's still the best partner I ever had. Oliver, a Belgian guy, was equally good on scene, but Oliver didn't know the region as well, and didn't have Cliff's contacts in the fire and sheriff's departments, or Cliff's driving skill, as Cliff started his career as a policeman. Cliff liked to slide the rig around turns. Cops get a lot more training and experience driving fast than we do. I can remember responding hot to a call once, riding the governor at 93 mph, only to have two black Dodge Chargers whip by, doing at least 120. Couple cops teasing us.

Still, one of the most brilliant saves I ever saw accomplished was, actually, on a transport call, which is why it's in this book instead of in *Earn Money Sleeping*.

It was a BLS transport, taking a patient from a sniff (SNF: Specialized Nursing Facility) to an emergency room to be seen for an infection or something.

When I went into the patient's room, I could see that not only was she sleeping deeply, but she had a very reduced sensorium. Barely conscious at best.

I also noticed that I really had to pee.

Now, we are not supposed to use the patient's bathroom, and always supposed to be on our best behavior in facilities, which must be encouraged to call our service at all times for all their transports. But in this case, I was way down at the other end of the hall from the nursing station, it was a facility new to me, so I didn't know where the staff bathroom was, and surely the patient was not going to notice anything, so I slipped into the patient's bathroom.

Much to my horror, when I got out, there was the RN, standing in the middle of the patient's room. And glaring at me to boot.

"Do you always use the patient's bathroom?" she snarled.

"No, not at all," I said sheepishly.

Well, I think it's inappropriate," she went on. "Unacceptable."

I kind of slunk off. I thought she was overdoing it, but I couldn't think of anything mollifying to say. "Not as unacceptable as sexually harassing strange men about their bathroom habits" didn't seem like it would help.

What I found out later was that my partner, Doug, went into the room just after me, when the nurse was still fuming, and still contemplating calling in a complaint. She brought up the bathroom incident and my unseemly behavior to Doug as soon as she caught sight of him.

Without missing a beat, quick as a flash, with his catlike reflexes, Doug said, smoothly, "Well," looking around circumspectly, "he's that age, you know?"

"What do you mean?"

"You know, at a certain age men start getting some problems, with, you know, with their, well, prostates, you know."

"Oh," she said, guilelessly.

"Well, don't tell him I said anything, please," Doug said, looking around guiltily.

"No, of course not," she whispered.

Now that's what I call having your back.

GOOD SPORT

Before I tell this next story, I have to explain the Glasgow Coma Score for lay readers. Sorry.

For readers interested in technical writing problems, I might mention that this is a problem I have not been able to find a solution for. I believe there is no solution. That is, in order to understand stories about what happens during EMS calls, you need to know a few medical facts, abbreviations and names of conditions.

Explaining them in a glossary is no good, because many readers will never consult a glossary. Explaining them once at the beginning of a book is no good because people forget or maybe even skip that section. It's particularly no good with kindle and e-texts because it's hard to jump around to glossaries, tables of contents etc.

This is one of the ways a physical book is still better than an e text. That is, indeed, the thing with most technical innovations. They may be improvements in many ways, and yet you lose some qualities. It's kind of like taking Coumadin when you have an irregular heartbeat. Yes, it will help prevent strokes and heart attacks, but it will also cause a lot of other problems, hopefully not as severe or prevalent.

Anyway, it's also no good to keep explaining the term every time it comes up. It hopelessly slows down the story, and turns off and bores all the readers who do know or remember what the term means, which may indeed be the majority of the readers of a book on EMS.

You would think the solution would be simple. A mere tap on your phone or computer or pad will get you a nice wiki or google explanation of any word or abbreviation you care to know about. But that seems not to satisfy a lot of armchair critics either. You lazy fools! Why am I doing all the work?

Sorry. Let's get back to the point. The Glasgow Coma Score, or GCS, is a rating system to describe a patient's mental status or depth of unconsciousness. Just saying someone is comatose or 'not responding' doesn't say much. Particularly when you consider that for EMS or ER staff, "unresponsive" means GCS 3, no response of any kind to any stimulus; whereas to a nursing home caretaker, it often seems to mean, "Mary isn't talking much today." Which can be a significant finding, but not what we would call unresponsive, when we are responding with lights and sirens.

GCS score is based on three categories.

The first is eye opening. No response gets you 1 point; to pain, 2; to speech, 3; spontaneously, 4.

Next is verbal response. No vocalization gets you 1 point, moans or grunts or incomprehensible speech gets you 2, inappropriate words gets you 3, confused gets you 4, and fully oriented gets you 5. Inappropriate doesn't mean they hit on you or make racist or sexist remarks. It means that if you ask someone what year it is, and they say 1989, that's confused. If they say Eggplant Parmesan, that's inappropriate.

New partners often get confused themselves when I reply to incomprehensible speech from a dementia patient by saying "Richard Nixon."

They say, "What?"

I say, "Wasn't he asking me who the 30th president of the US was?"

The last category is Motor. No response, no reflex action, nothing, is 1. Decerebrate extension, convulsively spreading out the arms and legs and arching the back, is 2. This is also called decerebrate posturing and occurs after a head injury, if the brain stem is being pushed down into the spinal opening by swelling of the brain, which has few places to go in the skull. Next, flexion, or decorticate posturing, is pulling the arms into the body. That's 3. Bad but not as bad. Withdraws from Pain is 4. Painful stimulus causes the patient to withdraw generally, not just the affected, say, finger. Localizes pain is 5. Obeys commands is 6.

These are not always easy to tell apart and are not equally relevant for trauma or medical or chronic conditions. It's sometimes hard to tell if someone is 3, 4 or 5. Usually you're not more than one off, though, and of course these conditions can improve or worsen or reverse direction.

However, this is still the best quick way to determine a patient's level of responsiveness, and it is used by all medical personnel in or out of hospital.

But here are some of the problems. Suppose your patient speaks Hungarian. He's incomprehensible to you, but he could be a genius in Hungarian. Suppose he's perfectly alert and oriented, but he doesn't feel like talking to you for one reason or another. Maybe because you keep saying Richard Nixon whenever he asks you something. Supposing he has dysarthria, and cannot move his tongue or mouth adequately, but in his head he's perfectly alert and oriented. Suppose he's mute or deaf. Even if he looks like he's making sense, in a language you know a little, still, unless you are fluent, you can't tell if he's confused or not.

Suppose he's blind but otherwise perfectly normal. No eye opening, but he's not altered mental at all.

It doesn't work for psych patients very well either. She can answer your four questions about where she is, what her name is, what year it is, and what's going on perfectly well, but she is still convinced alien insects have crawled into her ears and are taking over her brain.

As far as obeying commands, maybe he doesn't want to. Maybe he doesn't withdraw from pain because he is faking unconsciousness. It may be surprising but patients fake seizures and unconsciousness on such a regular basis that crews see faked seizures more often than real ones, which have usually subsided by the time crews get there.

And this too is more complex than first appears. A pseudo seizure or faked unconsciousness still isn't normal, and does indicate altered mental status of some kind.

For some reason, you get a lot of adolescent women who appear more comatose than they really are. I think they may be the same ones who used to swoon in the 19th century.

In fact, we carry an instrument which I believe is designed for just this purpose. It's called a nasal trumpet. It's a rubber, horn shaped thing which comes in various sizes and lengths. Supposedly you measure from corner of ear to corner of mouth, select that length trumpet, and insert it in the nose of an unconscious person, to help her breathe better. So she won't gag on her own tongue, which, believe it or not, is the main reason unconscious people can't breathe, including those with sleep apnea.

It is, however, perfectly useless for this purpose. That is, if you shove it up the nose of a deeply unconscious person, nothing at all happens. You can't convince me it's helping him breathe. Unlike an oral airway, a J tube, which is the right instrument, till you intubate.

However, and this is what we do use it for, if you shove it up someone's nose and they are conscious, they immediately sit up, start gagging and snorting, and try to pull the thing out of their nose. Try it, you'll see.

It's also really entertaining. In large part because it's scary when a patient is deeply unconscious and you can't figure out why. Seeing them sit up, gag and snort, well, it seems like they deserve it for faking something just to scare you and their loved ones. Almost anyone would rather observe a rhino imitation than work a full arrest.

With some experience, though, you don't really care why they are unconscious, as soon as you have reliably ascertained that they are medically stable. If the patient's heart rate and rhythm are good, vitals are fine, color, muscle tone, blood sugar all check out, if his pupils are equal, round and reactive, neither excessively dilated nor pinpoint (or if you can't see them because he's rolling them up in his head to avoid you), he's warm, pink and dry, then he can be unconscious all he likes. Let the ER figure it out. That's why they make the big bucks.

For example, I remember a 16 year old girl we found on a couch, unconscious, after her family called us in a panic. Her color, vitals, muscle tone, the way she was holding her face all looked fine to me, so even before I looked at her blood sugar and put her on a monitor, I leaned in close to her, and said,

"You have to answer 3 questions for me or I have to stick a tube down your throat to make sure you can breathe right."

This was perfectly legit. The rule is, Glasgow eight, intubate, though actually I usually won't intubate someone, at least right away, who has an intact gag reflex. The point is, you have to protect the airway from aspirating vomit. ABC. Airway Breathing Circulation.

I said, "Where are you?"

"At home," she whispered, eyes closed.

"What's your name?"

"Jessica."

"What year is it?"

"2014."

"OK. I won't bother you again."

Because this TV thing where someone says "Talk to me, stay with me, hang in there buddy etc" is pointless. Keeping someone talking or awake or whatever is not doing anything to help them, except perhaps in the case where they have taken an overdose of opiates and you're trying to get them to exert themselves so they can circulate blood and excrete the drug before going completely unconscious. Even then, for us, some Narcan or other expedients will work better. Let them snooze or do whatever it is they are doing. If I have them hooked up to a monitor I can get a much better idea of where they are than by what they say or do.

I turned to her parents and said, "Did you hear?"

"Yes," the alarmed father said, "but she's not normal. She's never acted like this before."

"I understand. We're going to take her to the hospital right now. I just wanted to reassure you a little about her condition; she's not going to die."

And sure enough, psych disorders are medical conditions and do require EMS. But unless you have a weapon or means of suicide handy, psych just won't kill you right away, even though the long term morbidity and mortality of major depression or psychosis or bipolar disorder are worse than pneumonia or a femur fracture.

So, now we got that all cleared away, this time we're taking a terminal patient on hospice back home to die. He has end stage cardiac disease. He has a DNR, otherwise he ought to stay in the ICU, obviously, because he's bad and only going to get worse.

Pretty bad already. His heart rate and rhythm are all right but he's breathing at 4 a minute where 8 to 20 is normal. When he's breathing at all. He also has apneic periods. He's not doing the Cheyne Stokes thing where he has apnea, then breathes faster and faster, then slower and slower, then apnea again. Very weird terminal breathing pattern. You also see neurogenic breathing, which is rapid and deep but kind of autonomous, not related to anything external, invariable. It usually means oxygen is circulating but isn't being used by the body. There's also agonal breathing, known as guppy breathing in EMS speech. Cyanosis is smurf.

His blood pressure is 68/40. This is not normal for anyone, but particularly not for a guy who lists at 250 lbs, like this dude. And actually probably weighs more, because he has huge amounts of fluid everywhere, owing to his heart and kidneys being unable to excrete it.

He's also a GCS 3, which is going to be the point of this story. No response to anything. Vegetative, if it lasts.

The nurse, 50-ish, smart, articulate, kind of beautiful, thinks he should just die in the hospital, or not have been brought there in the first place. Because all of us are not sure he will even make it home. Particularly since, being hospice, he's been taken off all the meds which were keeping him going.

The RN and I were talking about hospice while my partner was getting his paperwork together. We both like it, but she was stricter about it. I was telling her the dehydration story about my mom, told in my hospice section, and she was sympathetic to the hospice position.

"By then, it should only be about comfort," she said.

"Yeah but dehydration isn't comfortable, and my mom was fully alert and oriented, she should still be in charge of her own care. I mean it wasn't like we wanted chemo or surgery."

"True, those are the tough ones. You like your hospice patients to be deadly sick and comatose."

"How far is his home?" she asks. "Maybe you can go fast."

"Yeah," I say. "Lights and sirens. Code three hospice transport."

She smiles. Very nice smile.

We are not in any hurry, actually. With a DNR, we can drop him off dead or alive. She needn't worry about us leaving him behind. My partner is a marine.

Actually, he's a big, blond, young, goodlooking fireman with long hair sticking out of his cap, and a good sense of humor. Lively, energetic guy who swears a lot. I get along with him very well. Makes for a really pleasant shift, even though we're running our butts off, getting contradictory messages on our pager, and being yelled at over the phone by our boss. "Yes ma'am."

"I hate this fucking job," he likes to say. He's into fire and EMS, not this transport service he's doing only for extra money.

So many firemen and medics do their 24 on/48 off and then pick up 2 or even more shifts a week elsewhere. 80 hours a week. Good money but crazy. When do they exercise, see their kids, wives, cook? Often they don't.

Well, we get to our patient's house without incident. He is holding his blood oxygen SATs (saturation) on oxygen via nonrebreather mask (NRB), despite hardly breathing. Amazing how little air the body really needs at rest. Though we are quintupling the amount of O2 he's getting, compared to room air. This is equivalent, roughly, to him breathing five times as often. Room air is 21% O2, every liter you add via oxygen device is 3% more. If the bag on the NRB is full, he's breathing 100% O2. In his case, this just takes 8 liters, because he's barely using it.

It's a nice little house in a green suburban neighborhood all decked out for the great spring we are having. A big tree has split, laying half of itself on his lawn. An ash. Usually strong trees. It strikes me as a poetic echo, since I assume, naturally, that it happened recently, just about the time the master went terminal. But no, I see later that attempts have been made, via chain, already gone rusty, to keep it from splitting further, and that the branches occluding the driveway have been pruned off. To what end, I'm not sure, because now they have half a tree lying in their front yard. But that turns out to be poetic echoing too, as you will see.

So the hospice RN (LVN?) nurse meets us at the truck. She's enthusiastic and motivated but also kind of naive. Actually kind of clueless, it turns out, but we appreciate her attitude.

"He's imminent," I say, after we exchange greetings.

"Oh," she says. "Better get him in quick. We wouldn't want him to die on the driveway!"

I'm kind of feeling askance by now, because this is starting to get odd. I mean, what, we would dump him in the driveway, and say, "Our work here is done."? He's going inside for his family to say goodbye anyway. And, at a Glasgow 3, it isn't going to make any difference to him anymore where he dies.

"Oh," she says, "it's really sad. His wife lost her sister and her aunt this same year."

"Wow," I say. "That's really tough. And their tree too."

She looks at the tree but she isn't following.

As we are getting him inside, which is a bit of a production, since we have to jog the stretcher off road onto the lawn to get around the tree ("engage the four wheel drive, sir!"), and then collapse the stretcher, and sit him up, to get around the corner, past his front door, to the bed in the living room. I'm really glad the stretcher makes it, because carrying a 250 pound plus guy around corners, even with a strapping fireman to help you, is no joke. Miss LVN is light weight in more sense than one, too.

Meanwhile, she's talking to him.

"My name is Janice, I'll be taking care of you, and this is Freda, your regular caregiver, do you remember her?"

"He's a GCS 3," I say.

The LVN hands me a blank look. All right, hospice staff person—I'm starting to doubt she's even an LVN, much less RN. What RN doesn't know the Glasgow Coma Scale? In fact, she appears never to have heard of it. I'd look at her badge, but I'm busy. And I don't really care.

"How are you feeling?" she asks him. "Is there something we can do for you to make you more comfortable?"

De Tarbaby, he don' say nuffin.

"Which ear is he deaf in?" she asks. "I heard he's really hard of hearing."

"Yeah, he is," I say.

But she's still talking to him. "I bet you're glad to be home at last! We'll get you settled in your bed!"

De Tarbaby, he don' say nuffin.

Now it's possible people in deep comas can hear and understand some things, or at least respond neurologically to voices in some way. I kind of doubt it. But let her do her thing. She's engaged, warmhearted and enthusiastic. In some ways, personality can make up for brains.

We have to manipulate him quite a bit to sit him up so as to get the stretcher collapsed to round the corner, and then to get him sitting up in position on the bed. Unfortunately I whack his arm pretty hard on the bed railing pulling him up, because he's so heavy and his arm is so lifeless and floppy. I try to be careful, but things happen. This would be grisly if we weren't so used to it. Fortunately, family isn't nearby. The hospice lady was making it all seem like "My weekend with Bernie," though.

I touch his eyes in front of her, so she can see what I'm talking about. He doesn't blink or flinch or move in any way. Doesn't ever, for any reason. GCS 3.

"Oh, he's such a good sport!" she says. "He never complains!"

We help her arrange him, which she's grateful for, because she's heard we're not allowed to get sheets and dirty mats out from under him, sit him up, position him etc. once we've delivered him. I don't know if that's true or not. It might be a liability issue. But we always do.

"Oh, you're such good sport," she says to him.

De Tarbaby, he don' say nuffin.

"No," I say, "don't worry about it. We're here to help; we're in your service."

So after thanks and goodbyes and signature, we work our way around the tree with our stretcher and back to the ambulance. Neill looks around to make sure we're out of earshot, and starts laughing.

"Yeah," I say. "I want that on my tombstone. He was such a good sport."

"You can't make this stuff up," he says.

"They can say, 'well, he was a real asshole while he was alive, a total whiner, always pissing and moaning about one thing and another, but after he died, he was such a good sport.'"

"Yeah, you could kick him or throw dirt on him or whatever and he never complained."

"So, sport, on to the next call?"

Which happened to be another Basic discharge, taking a dementia patient back to his Memory Care nursing home unit from the hospital, where he had gone for some respiratory problems.

This was a totally different kind of patient. He was medically stable, in reasonable general health, despite some chronic conditions. Most AD—Alzheimer--patients have serious chronic illnesses, but not infrequently you run into one who is healthy as a horse, just demented. They are hardly ever nice, happy old ladies who are just a little confused, and neither would you be if your brain was falling apart. He was hard to arouse at first, kind of lethargic, but by the time we got him home, he was sitting up, looking around, warm, pink and dry, vital signs stable etc.

He was also profoundly demented. He never said a word or made a sound. He had that stiff blank look on his face, and it was pretty clear that while he was kind of generally aware of his surroundings, he really had no idea where he was, who we were or what was happening, and what we said to him meant nothing. He was not paying attention, as it were.

Fortunately this was not making him unbearably anxious, as it would most people, especially when you consider that the short term memory loss means they can't get used to it. Everything that hurts comes as a new unpleasant surprise every five minutes.

Well, we had some trouble accessing his nursing home, which was concerning only because the boss was still riding us about our on scene and destination times. We were getting pages, several at a time, even when still occupied with a patient. She was saying, "I told you to check your pager when it goes off!"

It was going off seemingly by the minute, though. "Yes ma'am," I said. "Sorry." What I wanted to say, was, 'Sorry, the pager is so hot I was afraid to touch it.'

There's also my Porsche transmission/brain focus issue, aka, it's hard for me to walk and chew gum at the same time. If I'm focused on one thing, like a patient, my brain tends to ignore other things, like hysterical pagers. One patient at a time, please.

Multi-tasking is overrated. Usually it means someone is doing four things badly, instead of one well. I remember a partner sitting on our couch at the station, watching TV, texting, talking on the phone and listening to her I-pod all at the same time.

"I can't believe you're doing all that at once," I said.

"Yeah, I'm really good at multi-tasking," she said.

"Technically, I think to call it multi-tasking, at least one of them has to be an actual task," I said. "You're multi-entertaining. AKA ADHD."

This nursing home is Kafkaesque. It's not a bad place, though it is the one where the enraged, demented resident seized the fire extinguisher, backed into a corner and held off several staffers with it. We transported the nurse who was covered in fire suppressant powder. I already told that story.

But whichever entrance you approached, it was always the wrong one. Besides the front, there were two in the back and one on the side. We already had gotten a page stating we should not use the main, royal entrance. The porte cochere and beautifully appointed foyer were for paying guests, not waste management and other service personnel. This was an automatic page which always went out whenever a crew was sent to this facility. Because saying, "I'm sorry, I'll never do it again," didn't seem to serve, when you came in the front door, like at any other nursing home. I had tried it several times, and they seemed to doubt my sincerity, for some reason. Every time. Maybe I didn't look sorry.

To cover my ass, I asked dispatch, when I called destination, which entrance the facility wanted us to use. So if I went to the wrong one or took extra time finding the right one, I would have an excuse.

The boss, still on the radio, alas, said, "The side one."

Well, as described, there are three side entrances, but I wasn't going to get into a discussion on the radio about the facility floor plan. Boss was already loaded for bear. She would rightfully have considered we could figure this out without her micromanaging us from across town over the radio. She probably had never even been there before, anyway. Which was all true enough, but the whole issue wouldn't have arisen if she wasn't micromanaging us to start with.

Our boss is cool. She's a loud, colorful, six foot redhead who is kind and extremely intelligent. She's built up a multi-million dollar ambulance transport corporation from scratch. She also has a really short fuse, and no hesitation whatsoever about telling all and sundry what's on her mind. Blind Trust is not her operating principle, and that position is well taken, usually. She's always right because she usually is.

I was walking down the corridor at HQ after shift one evening when I ran into her coming the other way. I hadn't laid eyes on her for a while. In the old days you had more contact with her, but her business has gotten really big. Not a mom and pop any more, but the major provider for a city of 2 million.

So we greeted each other enthusiastically.

"I really like that new picture of yourself you put up by the checkout," I said.

Confused, she looked at the checkout computer in the corner. On the wall next to it was a motivational poster, labelled Pride, which was a picture of a lion. It looked like it was having a good day. Which for a lion means it had either just eaten someone or was planning to.

She blushed and started laughing. She's great. You do want to stay out of her way most of the time though. Lioness is definitely her totem animal.

Anyway, back to the Alzheimer's unit. Getting into a locked ward is always a chore. Usually, after you obtain entry to the premises, as the cops call it, you eventually run into a staffer who will tell you the door code. Rarely, the receptionist will tell you, if there is one, but their main function is to guard the bathroom key. So you punch in the code, get the stretcher through the door, line up the stretcher and bed, lift the patient onto the bed via drawsheet, get the paperwork signed, hand over the packet and patient possessions, joke around with the nurses if they are cute, clean the stretcher, re-sheet it, and then you head back to the locked door, after maybe ten minutes or more.

Do you remember the code? If so, you pass.

If not, you can search for a staffer. But, given that most of these facilities are understaffed, it usually appears that no one works there. Of course, there are plenty of helpful, demented patients around, with nothing else to do. You could ask one of them for the exit code. Start by explaining what a code is. But no staff to be seen. Certainly no one who has time to help able bodied and supposedly alert and oriented medics exit. Besides, perhaps being unable to remember a 5 digit code for ten minutes (no excuse that you're kind of busy) is a sign that a couple days in Memory Care will do you a lot of good. After some bingo, wheelchair exercise sessions, 40's movies and sing-alongs, a few tabs of Namenda, you'll be ready for the truck again!

If you can get someone to come pick you up, because the nurses won't let you have a phone, even if you remember how to use one. And anyway taxi services know better than to respond to that address.

You could call 911, like the patient in the Methodist ER. "OK, chest pain," the dispatcher said. "Where are you? You're where? Well, even if we did come and get you, where would we bring you? Oh, any other ER."

"Yeah, they're not helping me here." True story.

But at this Rehab facility, aka nursing home, we hadn't even got in yet. I banged on the side door, which had a sign saying, "Emergency entrance only. All patients and visitors use the main entrance." Well, all the doors except the main entrance had that same sign. And we had been explicitly told not to use the main entrance, unlike at every other nursing home. Besides, we ARE an emergency service. Even if this was no emergency.

A grumpy looking, overweight individual noticed me, after someone else pointed us out, and walked the length of the long corridor to my door. He pointed to the sign above the door when he got there. The walk hadn't done him any good, apparently.

He was kind enough to actually open it to talk to me, though.

"Sorry," I said. "Which door would you like us to use? I never can figure it out."

"The one in the back," he says.

"Which one in the back? The one in that corner or the one all the way around?" I said, pointing.

"The one all the way around," he said.

"All right, thank you."

"OK you're welcome." They did seem to be cheerful today at least.

I got back in the driver's seat of the rig. I had not been dumb enough to unload the patient yet, and Neill was waiting patiently in the back with him.

I drove around the building to the appropriate door. This procedure, by the way, is way less amusing when there is an emergency we are responding to, rather than just delivering a stable patient.

We unloaded.

"This does not mean they are actually going to let us in," I said. "I've been here before."

But they did. Without banging and knocking or trying out various likely codes on the doorpad. Three cheerful and charming young ladies.

They were in good moods too. Things were looking up.

"Sorry," we said. "I never know which entrance to come in."

"Well," one said, "the one nearest the patient's room."

"I don't really know the layout of your facility though."

"That's true," she said, generously giving me the benefit of the doubt. Can't expect every medic to be the sharpest knife in the drawer.

We trundled our patient through the locked dementia ward doors to his fine new room. Everyone was very enthusiastic. Staff was welcoming the patient, saying "We're glad to have you back, Mr Stevens"etc.

Tarbaby he don' say nuffin.

"Wow," I said, joining in the fun. "Great room. Huge. The royal suite! Still got that new room smell."

"Yeah, freshly painted," they said, proudly. Place did look nice, and having three staffers accompanying you does indicate adequate staffing, which is always the big problem for nursing homes. "You're going to love it, aren't you, Mr. Stevens?"

Tarbaby he don' say nuffin.

We lined up the stretcher to move the patient.

"Is this his usual mental status?" I asked. "Does he talk? He hasn't for us."

"No, this is the way he is. He doesn't have much to say."

"But he's a good sport," I said.

Neill did not look at me.

"Oh yeah, he's a good sport! Aren't you, Mr. Stevens?"

Tarbaby he don' say nuffin.

We get him in the bed and head for the exit. We have not been confided what the code is to get out, but this time, unusually, a staffer is clever enough to realize, having had this happen daily, that we are not going to be able to get out through the locked door without the code, and so he accompanies us. Memory Care units are locked to prevent elopement, which is the correct locution, actually. Not infrequently there is some devious old dude hanging about the entrance, feebly trying to effectuate an escape. In his wheelchair. Breaks my heart to abandon him.

Every time this happens, I imagine a staffer coming up to me, when I'm trying to get out, and saying, "Sir, sir, you go back to your room now, sir."

"But I'm a paramedic."

"Sir, you used to be a paramedic. You need to get back to your room now. You don't want us to have to sedate you like last time, do you?"

This time we get out unscathed though.

"So, see, I told you stealing these uniforms would work," I say.

"Those poor medics we swapped clothes with," Neill says. "I wonder if they will ever get out."

"I hope they're good sports."

POSTSCRIPT

This is the last of a series of three books on my experiences as a field paramedic. Unless I feel like writing another one, or there is a huge public outcry and demand. All three are written in short pieces describing individual calls or grouped calls.

For those of you interested in writing, as such, I can add here, to my discussion above about medical vocabulary, a few notes about style and approach.

I grew up on the traditions of the realistic novel as it has been written for a couple hundred years, often if not always containing long descriptions of people, scenes, surrounding details and even inconsequential extra dialogue to establish a sense of felt life. Often there is quite a lot of subtle psychology or philosophy too. I've been greatly moved by many of these novels, but the genre has become to some extent exhausted for me. One of them has to be unusually intelligent or different in an interesting way to catch my attention now, or has to be about a subject or group of people who fascinate me particularly.

So I've chosen a more stripped down form of narrative, for several reasons, actually.

First, I want to write mostly in the demotic American of the street, the language spoken by the medics I work with.

I want a medic to be able to read these stories without getting bored or bogged down in any excesses of description, commentary, psychology. Besides, subtle psychological issues tend to go over my head a lot anyway, especially when I am not paying attention, like when on scene. Most people aren't all that subtle most of the time.

Then, I've noticed that both historically and in daily life, people do not tell stories in the way realistic novelists do. You find little of that stuff in Homer, the Bible, Chaucer, Dante or in fablieau or Herodotus or the Decameron. Even during the height of the realistic novel you find writers like Babel cutting to the bone, using periods like cannonballs.

It was a huge esthetic breakthrough to find out what Mme Bovary was thinking, to see Leopold Bloom taking a bath or eating a pork kidney. Or to follow Swann's excruciating obsessing over Odette.

But do we really want to know what everyone is thinking all the time, or watch people eating, or itch our way through all their obsessions? If so, there's always the Internet.

And in daily life, no one has ever told stories like a realistic novelist. You say, "Do you know what happened to me at work today? Well, Joe, the guy who sits next to me, the one with the bad temper" and then you just get to the point of the story. You don't go into what he was wearing and eating and thinking unless one of those is the point.

So besides writing in the demotic, I've chosen to get to the point. Probably the language is still too complex, and I do have a weakness for humorous observations, in other writers as well as my own work.

This seemed appropriate for the world of EMS. The platinum ten minutes and the golden hour can be guidelines for writers too. Airway Breathing Circulation Diesel.